# Multiple Choice Q...
# MEDICINE, SURGERY A...

**Modern Nursing Series**

*General Editors*

A. J. Harding Rains, MS, FRCS
Professor of Surgery, Charing Cross Hospital Medical School, Honorary Consultant Surgeon to the Army
Miss Valerie Hunt, SRN, SCM, OND, RNT
Formerly District Nursing Officer, Avon Area Health Authority (Teaching), Member General Nursing Council of England and Wales
Miss Susan E. Norman, SRN, NDNCert, RNT
Nurse Tutor, The Nightingale School, St Thomas's Hospital, London

---

Some titles in the Series which are available as paperbacks. A complete list can be obtained from the publisher.

**Textbook of Medicine
with relevant physiology and anatomy**
R. J. Harrison

**Microbiology in Patient Care**
H. I. Winner

**Obstetrics and Gynaecology**
Joan M. E. Quixley
Michael D. Cameron

**Venereology and Genito-Urinary Medicine**
R. D. Catterall

**Revision Notes on Psychiatry**
K. T. Koshy

**Principles of Surgery and Surgical Nursing**
Selwyn Taylor

**Principles of Medicine and Medical Nursing**
J. C. Houston and
Hilary Hyde White

**Rheumatology**
D. R. Swinson and
W. R. Swinburn

**Vascular Surgery**
R. E. Horton

# Multiple Choice Questions and Answers with explanatory notes on
# MEDICINE, SURGERY AND NURSING
## including relevant physiology and anatomy

R. J. Harrison Ch.B., MD

*Lecturer in Medicine for the St. Helens and Knowsley Area Health Authority. Examiner for the General Nursing Council for England and Wales, 1961–1970*

HODDER AND STOUGHTON
LONDON SYDNEY AUCKLAND TORONTO

British Library Cataloguing in Publication Data

Harrison, R. J.
 Multiple choice questions and answers
 with explanatory notes on medicine, surgery
 and nursing including relevant physiology
 and anatomy. – (Modern nursing series)
 1. Medicine – Problems, exercises, etc.
 2. Nursing
 I. Title  II. Series
 610.73     RT55

ISBN 0 340 24707 X

First published 1981

Copyright © 1981 R. J. Harrison

All Rights Reserved. No part of this publication may be reproduced or transmitted in any form or by any means, electronic or mechanical, including photocopy, recording, or any information storage and retrieval system, without permission in writing from the publisher.

Printed in Great Britain for
Hodder and Stoughton Educational,
a division of Hodder and Stoughton Limited,
Mill Road, Dunton Green, Sevenoaks, Kent
by Biddles Ltd, Guildford, Surrey

# Preface

Multiple choice questions are one type of objective testing used by examining bodies, such as the General Nursing Council, the Professional and Linguistic Association Board of the General Medical Council, the Colleges and the Universities, as part of their written examinations. Multiple choice questions eliminate any possible examiner bias from the marking. They can reveal the student's judgement as well as his factual knowledge.

Another type of test is the matching-block question, some examples of which are given at the end of this book.

Some multiple choice questions appear to be ambiguous or confusing. In this book, therefore, each solution is explained so that the student can see *how* it has been arrived at. Most of these answers includes more than the one piece of information required as a solution to the question, so that the book may be used, not only for practice in answering multiple choice questions, but also as an aid to the revision of the subject.

Further details of a particular disorder can be obtained by reading the appropriate section in *Textbook of Medicine, with relevant physiology and anatomy*, by R. J. Harrison (Unibooks, Hodder and Stoughton). It may be used in conjunction with this book, which is likely to be especially useful in the few months prior to sitting the examination question papers.

# Contents

482 multiple choice questions and answers in medicine, surgery and nursing, including related physiology and anatomy.

Questions are grouped into sections, each section containing an average of approximately 30 questions and answers. Explanations are also given where appropriate.

Ten matching-block questions and answers are given at the end of the book.

|   |   | Page |
|---|---|---|
| Preface | | v |
| Contents | | vi |
| Multiple Choice Questions—Method | | viii |
| 1 General questions | 10 questions | 1 |
| Answers | | 2 |
| 2 Nutrition | 17 questions | 3 |
| Answers | | 5 |
| 3 Water, electrolytes, and acid-base balance | 12 questions | 6 |
| Answers | | 8 |
| 4 Immunity and infection | 24 questions | 10 |
| Answers | | 13 |
| 5 Blood and lymphoreticular system | 26 questions | 15 |
| Answers | | 18 |
| 6 Cardiovascular system | 46 questions | 21 |
| Answers | | 27 |
| 7 Respiratory system | 33 questions | 32 |
| Answers | | 36 |
| 8 Digestive system, part 1 | 33 questions | 39 |
| part 2 | 46 questions | 43 |
| Answers | | 49 |
| 9 Liver and biliary system | 32 questions | 55 |
| Answers | | 59 |
| 10 Urinary system | 52 questions | 62 |
| Answers | | 69 |
| 11 Reproductive system | 19 questions | 73 |
| Answers | | 75 |

# Contents

| | | |
|---|---|---|
| 12 Endocrine system | 43 questions | 77 |
| Answers | | 82 |
| 13 Nervous system | 43 questions | 86 |
| Answers | | 91 |
| 14 Musculoskeletal system and skin | 28 questions | 94 |
| Answers | | 97 |
| 15 The special senses and geriatrics | 18 questions | 100 |
| Answers | | 102 |
| Matching block questions | 10 questions | 104 |
| Answers | | 106 |

# Multiple Choice Questions—Method

Questions should not be read until the subject matter has been learned thoroughly from other sources, such as textbooks.

All the questions in one section should be answered, without stopping, before checking your answers with those at the end of the section. If you have answered a question incorrectly it would be advisable to revise the appropriate section in the textbook(s).

Each question is followed by four possible answers only ONE of which is correct. The correct answer should be underlined. If you change your mind, cross out the incorrectly underlined answer and underline your new choice, e.g.:

(a), (b), (c), (d); changed to (a), (b̶), (c), (d).

Alternatively, the answers may be jotted down on a separate sheet of paper.

One mark is given for a correct answer, one mark is deducted for an incorrect answer and no mark is given or deducted for a question left unanswered. This method is used so that, in theory, those who guess should not gain any advantage, although in practice it is possible to make a lucky guess and gain by it.

The pass level is 50% of the maximum number of marks. For example, out of 33 questions in Chapter 7, the maximum number of marks is 33. If 22 are correctly answered, 3 are incorrectly answered and 8 are unanswered, the mark is 22 minus 3 (= 19), and $\frac{19}{33} \times 100 = 57\%$, which is a pass. On the other hand, if 20 are correctly answered, but 7 are incorrectly answered, and 6 are unanswered, the mark is 20 minus 7 (= 13), and $\frac{13}{33} \times 100 = 39\%$, which is a fail.

# 1 General Questions

1 Deep venous thrombosis is commonly caused by

   (a) taking anticoagulants   (b) drinking too much fluid
   (c) moving about in bed     (d) lying still in bed

2 Heredity is transmitted by

   (a) the prostate   (b) the uterus
   (c) genes         (d) electrolytes

3 A benign tumour of glandular cells is known as

   (a) adenoma   (b) osteoma
   (c) atheroma   (d) carcinoma

4 When a patient is to be given a drug, the most important item to check is

   (a) the patient's name   (b) the name of the drug
   (c) the dose of the drug
   (d) no one of these is more important than the others

5 Cancers are growths which

   (a) never spread to other parts of the body
   (b) are malignant
   (c) are not malignant   (d) never kill the patient

6 The concentration of isotonic saline is

   (a) 0.9%   (b) 2%   (c) 5%   (d) 10%

7 The concentration of isotonic dextrose is

   (a) 1%   (b) 5%   (c) 10%   (d) none of these

8 The normal number of chromosomes in the human is

   (a) 94   (b) 46   (c) 25   (d) 22

9 In cardiac arrest the most important immediate treatment is
   (a) oxygen     (b) adrenaline
   (c) to maintain respiration and the circulation
   (d) none of these

10 Shock may be due to
   (a) bleeding              (b) injury
   (c) pulmonary embolism    (d) any of these

# Answers

1 (d) Moving about in bed and anticoagulants help to prevent venous thrombosis
2 (c)
3 (a) The other tumours are of bone (osteoma) and malignant epithelium (carcinoma).
   Atheroma is a deposition of fatty material in arterial walls.
4 (d) *All* are important.
5 (b) Cancers are malignant and tend to spread and to kill the patient.
6 (a)
7 (b)
8 (b)
9 (c) Neither oxygen nor adrenaline are of any use if the circulation and respiration are absent.
10 (d)

# 2 Nutrition

1. Each day the average adult uses
   - (a) 2500 kcalories (10.5 MJ)
   - (b) 4500 kcalories (18.9 MJ)
   - (c) 1000 kcalories (4.2 MJ)
   - (d) 1500 kcalories (6.3 MJ)

2. Nitrogen is present in
   - (a) fat
   - (b) carbohydrate
   - (c) second class protein
   - (d) vitamin C

3. Nitrogen is not present in
   - (a) beef
   - (b) butter
   - (c) eggs
   - (d) chicken

4. The highest source of calcium is found in
   - (a) eggs
   - (b) rhubarb
   - (c) butter
   - (d) milk

5. Calcium is not of notable importance in
   - (a) bones
   - (b) teeth
   - (c) eyes
   - (d) blood clotting

6. Iron is not found in
   - (a) white sugar
   - (b) beef
   - (c) liver
   - (d) broad beans

7. Iodine is of prime importance in the formation of
   - (a) pyridoxine
   - (b) adrenaline
   - (c) bone
   - (d) thyroxine

8. Vitamin A is not required for
   - (a) vision in dim light
   - (b) bone growth
   - (c) healthy epithelium
   - (d) glomerular filtration

9. Thiamine (aneuryn, vitamin B1) deficiency causes
   - (a) cardiac failure in beri beri
   - (b) rickets
   - (c) 'night blindness'
   - (d) hypothyroidism

10 Riboflavin (vitamin B2) deficiency does not cause
   (a) stomatitis     (b) glossitis
   (c) polyneuritis   (d) dermatitis

11 Folic acid deficiency causes
   (a) dermatitis   (b) macrocytic anaemia
   (c) gout         (d) hypochromic anaemia

12 Vitamin B12 deficiency leads to
   (a) hypochromic anaemia   (b) macrocytic anaemia
   (c) microcytic anaemia    (d) aplastic anaemia

13 Vitamin C is not required for the formation of
   (a) antibodies   (b) red cells
   (c) saliva       (d) fibrous tissue

14 Vitamin C is not found in
   (a) fruit   (b) vegetables   (c) tomatoes   (d) meats

15 Vitamin D deficiency causes
   (a) renal calculi   (b) rickets or osteomalacia
   (c) gall stones     (d) pancreatitis

16 Vitamin K is required for the formation of
   (a) fibrinogen   (b) bile
   (c) platelets    (d) prothrombin

17 A low residue diet contains
   (a) baked custard, yoghourt, ice cream, white bread, potatoes, sugar, meat
   (b) brown bread, peas, beans, meat
   (c) radishes, cress, pickles, meat
   (d) onions, leeks, radishes, fruit, nuts, meat

# Answers

1. (a) Some people use more energy than others, e.g. a sedentary worker may use 2000 kcal or a coal miner 4000 kcal, but the *average* is 2500 kcal.
2. (c) Nitrogen is absent from fat, carbohydrate and vitamin C.
3. (b) All proteins contain nitrogen, e.g. beef, eggs, chicken.
4. (d)
5. (c) Calcium is essential in bones, teeth and blood clotting.
6. (a) White sugar is almost pure sucrose.
   Beef, liver and broad beans all contain iron.
7. (d) Thyroxine cannot be formed in the absence of iodine.
   Bone, like teeth, requires traces of *fluorine*.
8. (d) The glomerular filtrate is produced by the hydrostatic blood pressure.
   For health, a, b, and c all require vitamin A.
9. (a) The other deficiencies are vitamin D (rickets), vitamin A ('night blindness'), and thyroxine (hypothyroidism).
10. (c) Vitamin B2 deficiency causes stomatitis, glossitis and dermatitis.
11. (b) The red blood cells are large (macrocytes).
    Hypochromic anaemia is usually due to iron deficiency.
12. (b) The red cell precursors in the bone marrow are abnormally large (magaloblasts) and they produce large red cells (macrocytes), similar to those in folate deficiency.
    Aplastic anaemia is a failure of the bone marrow to produce cells.
13. (c) The question asks what vitamin C is *not* required for.
14. (d) Dietary lack of fresh fruit and vegetables leads to scurvy (vitamin C deficiency).
15. (b) Vitamin D deficiency causes rickets in children and osteomalacia in adults.
    Renal calculi and pancreatitis can be caused by an *excess* of vitamin D.
    Gall stones are usually due to precipitation of cholesterol from unstable solution in bile.
16. (d) Fibrinogen and platelets, although taking part in blood clotting, do not require vitamin K for their formation. Bile is needed for the absorption of fat-soluble vitamins such as vitamin K.
17. (a)

# 3 Water, Electrolytes, and Acid-base Balance

1 Which one of the following is not an electrolyte?
   (a) sodium       (b) potassium
   (c) phosphorus   (d) magnesium

2 Osmosis is the transfer, across a membrane, of
   (a) fluid into the compartment containing the weakest concentration of particles
   (b) fluid into the compartment containing the highest concentration of dissolved substances or particles
   (c) any substance, from a higher concentration to a lower one
   (d) fluid by hydrostatic pressure, from the compartment under higher pressure into that of lower pressure

3 Osmotic pressure is due to
   (a) all the particles in a liquid solution
   (b) some of the particles in a liquid solution
   (c) the blood pressure    (d) the plasma volume

4 In medicine, an isotonic solution is one which
   (a) contains sodium chloride    (b) contains dextrose
   (c) has the same osmotic pressure as urine
   (d) has the same osmotic pressure as plasma

5 The highest concentration of potassium is found in
   (a) cells     (b) plasma
   (c) urine     (d) cerebrospinal fluid

6 Which of the following is incorrect? Antidiuretic hormone
   (a) is released from the posterior part of the pituitary gland
   (b) increases the renal tubular re-absorption of water
   (c) increases plasma volume    (d) increases urine volume

# Water, Electrolytes, and Acid-base Balance

7 One of the following does not cause dehydration

   (a) water deficiency    (b) diabetic ketoacidotic coma
   (c) salt deficiency    (d) acute renal failure

8 One of the following does not cause oedema

   (a) hypoproteinaemia    (b) Addison's disease
   (c) congestive cardiac failure    (d) varicose veins

9 What is the total fluid loss from a normal adult in Britain in 24 hours?

   (a) 3.5 litres    (b) 2.5 litres
   (c) 1.5 litres    (d) 1.1 litres

10 Which of the following does not cause hyperkalaemia (high serum potassium)

   (a) acute renal failure    (b) haemolysis of red cells
   (c) a high cellular potassium    (d) Addison's disease

11 When 2.5 litres of intravenous fluid is to be administered in 24 hours

   (a) the procedure need not be explained to the patient
   (b) hyaluronidase may be used
   (c) the quantity of fluid given should be recorded
   (d) it should all be given as isotonic saline (0.9%) if the patient is not dehydrated

12 Unwanted excess of acid is excreted by

   (a) the lungs and kidneys    (b) the kidneys only
   (c) the liver and kidneys    (d) the liver only

# Answers

1. (c) Phos*phorus* is not an electrolyte and should not be confused with phos*phate*, which is.
   Electrolytes, e.g. sodium, potassium and magnesium, are substances which dissolve in water to form electrically charged particles (ions).
2. (b) Osmosis refers to the *transfer* of *fluid*, not the transfer of particles (it is likely to alter the *concentrations* of particles on each side of the membrane).
   (c) describes diffusion, (d) describes filtration.
3. (a) The blood pressure is a hydrostatic ('mechanical') pressure.
   Osmotic pressure is not *due to* the plasma volume, although it helps to maintain plasma volume by continuously 'sucking' tissue fluid into the blood capillaries.
4. (d) An isotonic solution may contain almost any substance, not just sodium chloride or dextrose, but it must have a concentration which is specific for that particular substance and which provides the same osmotic pressure as plasma, e.g. sodium chloride 0.9% or dextrose 5%, but *NOT*, e.g. dextrose 9% (which is hypertonic, i.e. stronger than isotonic).
5. (a) The potassium concentration in cells is thirty times that in plasma and urine, and forty times that found in CSF.
6. (d) Antidiuretic hormone, secreted by the pituitary, causes increased renal tubular re-absorption of water, thus increasing plasma volume and *decreasing* urine volume.
7. (d) In acute renal failure water fails to be excreted and is retained in the body.
8. (b) Cortisol and aldosterone stimulate the renal tubular cells to re-absorb salt and water from the tubular lumen. In Addison's disease (adrenal cortical failure) these are deficient, the kidneys, therefore, do not re-absorb as much salt and water and dehydration follows.
9. (b) The *total* loss in a temperate climate is 2.5 l. This includes urine (1.5 l), water vapour from the lungs (350 ml) and skin (500 ml), and faeces (150 ml).
10. (c) Acute renal failure leads to retention of potassium in the

# Water, Electrolytes, and Acid-base Balance

plasma. Cells, including red cells, contain large amounts of potassium, thus haemolysis releases potassium into the plasma (and gives a falsely high level). Potassium is retained in the plasma in Addison's disease owing partly to dehydration and partly to lack of adrenal corticosteroids which normally cause renal excretion of potassium in exchange for sodium.

11 (c) The procedure should be explained to the patient. Hyaluronidase is only used for subcutaneous, not intravenous, drips (it is seldom used now). If the patient is *not* dehydrated it is better to give saline 500 ml to dextrose 2 l otherwise the patient will be receiving too much salt.

12 (a) The lungs excrete carbonic acid, i.e. carbon dioxide and water vapour. The kidneys excrete non-volatile acids such as sulphuric and phosphoric acids. The liver does not excrete acid wastes.

# 4 Immunity and Infection

1 Body temperature is normally

   (a) higher in the rectum than in the mouth
   (b) higher in the axilla than in the mouth
   (c) higher in the mouth than in the rectum
   (d) 37.6° C

2 Using an ordinary glass and mercury thermometer under the tongue, the temperature is read after

   (a) 20 seconds         (b) 30 seconds
   (c) 30 to 60 seconds   (d) 2 to 5 minutes

3 Inflammation is not caused by

   (a) infection    (b) leucocytosis    (c) allergy    (d) injury

4 Immunity is not provided by

   (a) antibodies and lymphocytes    (b) vaccination
   (c) phagocytes                      (d) antibiotics

5 Neutrophil polymorphs do not

   (a) ingest bacteria      (b) digest bacteria
   (c) produce antibodies  (d) collect to form pus

6 Allergy is

   (a) an abnormal immune response    (b) bronchospasm
   (c) a normal immune response       (d) a skin rash

7 One of the following is incorrect. Antibodies are

   (a) produced by plasma cells    (b) immunoglobulins
   (c) produced by red cells
   (d) produced by lymphocytes

# Immunity and Infection

8 Autoimmune disease is due to

   (a) prednisolone   (b) antibodies produced by the body
   (c) antibodies produced by bacteria
   (d) vaccination

9 Micro-organisms which cause disease are called

   (a) pathogenic    (b) sporadic
   (c) endemic       (d) non-pathogenic

10 Micro-organisms may be spread by all except one of the following. Which is the exception?

   (a) droplets      (b) fomites
   (c) sterile dust  (d) ingestion

11 Staphylococci are often the cause of

   (a) tonsillitis   (b) boils   (c) cellulitis   (d) erysipelas

12 In rheumatic fever there is

   (a) infection of joint(s) with certain bacteria
   (b) bacterial myocarditis
   (c) preceding throat infection
   (d) bacterial infection in the skin nodules

13 Uncomplicated rheumatic fever is treated with rest in bed and

   (a) penicillin and soluble aspirin    (b) morphine
   (c) aspirin and restriction of fluids (d) gold ('Myocrisin')

14 One of the following is not a virus infection

   (a) influenza     (b) glandular fever
   (c) measles       (d) whooping cough

15 Which of the following is incorrect? Tuberculosis

   (a) commonly affects bone, lungs and lymph nodes
   (b) is common in immigrants
   (c) may be spread by dust or droplets
   (d) of the bovine type may be spread by pasteurised milk

16 Antituberculous drugs are usually given for

   (a) up to three weeks   (b) eight weeks
   (c) three months        (d) at least 9 months

17 A patient with pulmonary tuberculosis

   (a) need not be isolated if 'open' (sputum contains tubercle bacilli)
   (b) must always be treated in hospital
   (c) does not require a nutritious diet
   (d) must be notified to the Community Medical Officer

18 Bacillary dysentery is always treated with

   (a) antibiotic            (b) the patient in isolation
   (c) a high residue diet   (d) intravenous fluid

19 One of the following is untrue of leprosy. The tuberculoid type

   (a) produces a skin rash   (b) produces polyneuritis
   (c) is associated with low immunity
   (d) produces deformities

20 Gonorrhoea

   (a) infects millions of people in the world each year
   (b) does not spread outside the urethra
   (c) is not treated with antibiotic
   (d) is not transmitted at the same time as syphilis

21 Hydatid cysts develop from ova of a

   (a) canine tapeworm, *Taenia echinococcus*   (b) hookworm
   (c) beef tapeworm, *Taenia saginata*
   (d) dog roundworm, *Toxocara canis*

22 In an acute attack of malaria, symptoms are due to

   (a) rupture of red blood cells
   (b) toxins released by the parasite
   (c) the mosquito bite   (d) liver damage

# Immunity and Infection

23 The treatment of malarial parasites in the liver is

(a) chloroquine  (b) pyrimethamine
(c) primaquine  (d) amodiaquine

24 In tetanus infection the wound must be

(a) cleaned and sutured  (b) sterilised and sutured
(c) excised and sutured  (d) excised and left unsutured

# Answers

1 (a) The maximum normal temperature is 37.4° C in the rectum, 36.9° C in the mouth, and 36.7° C in the axilla.
2 (d) A falsely low recording may be obtained if read before 2 minutes.
3 (b) Infection, allergy and injury may all result in inflammation.
Leucocytosis may be a *result*, not a *cause*, of inflammation.
4 (d) Immunity is *intrinsic* resistance to infection. It is provided naturally by (a) and (c), and artificially by (b). Antibiotics may kill bacteria but are *extrinsic* agents.
5 (c) Polymorphs do *not* produce antibodies.
6 (a) The question asks for a definition of allergy, not the consequences of allergy (such as bronchospasm and skin rash).
7 (c) Antibodies are immunoglobulins and are produced by plasma cells and lymphocytes.
8 (b) In autoimmune disease the body produces antibodies against its own tissues.
Prednisolone is used as therapy. Bacteria liberate *antigens*, not antibodies.
Vaccination is irrelevant to the question.
9 (a) Patho = disease, genic = producing.
Sporadic and endemic refer, not to what micro-organisms *are*, but to how widespread is the disease they produce.

10 (c) *Sterile* dust does not contain living organisms.
11 (b) Tonsillitis, cellulitis and erysipelas are commonly due to haemolytic streptococci, not staphylococci.
12 (c) Joint and cardiac inflammation and skin nodules are due to autoimmune damage produced by the preceding throat infection, *not* to bacterial infection of these parts.
13 (a) Morphine should not be given. In cases uncomplicated by cardial failure, fluids should be given in abundance to compensate for sweating. Gold therapy is used in rheumatoid arthritis, not in rheumatic fever.
14 (d) Whooping cough is due to a bacillus, the others are virus infections.
15 (d) Pasteurisation kills tubercle bacilli.
16 (d) Recurrence is likely if the course of treatment is less than 9 months.
17 (d) The disease is notifiable. 'Open' means infectious, and therefore must be isolated. Mild or 'closed' (non-infectious) cases may be treated at home. All patients need good nutrition.
18 (b) Antibiotic is often not required. The diet should be low in residue.
Fluids may be adequate by mouth.
19 (c) Tuberculoid leprosy is associated with a high degree of immunity.
20 (a) It affects about 16 million people a year. It may spread locally, e.g. to epididymis or fallopian tubes, or systemically to joints, eye, heart etc.
Antibiotic should be given. Syphilis may be transmitted at the same time.
21 (a)
22 (a) Symptoms are due to haemolysis and anaemia.
23 (c)
24 (d)

# 5 Blood and Lymphoreticular System

1. Which one of the following is not a function of the plasma proteins?
   (a) haemostasis   (b) buffering of acids and bases
   (c) osmotic re-absorption of fluid from the interstitial tissues into the vascular system
   (d) to enable fluid to leave the vascular system by osmosis

2. The plasma of blood consists of
   (a) the fluid portion of clotted blood   (b) whole blood
   (c) the fluid portion of unclotted blood
   (d) blood without its protein

3. Which of the following is not a clotting factor in normal plasma?
   (a) prothrombin   (b) immunoglobulin
   (c) fibrinogen    (d) anti-haemophilic globulin

4. In the normal adult red and white blood cells are produced by
   (a) bone   (b) bone marrow   (c) liver   (d) spleen

5. The production of red blood cells in the marrow does not require
   (a) hydrochloric acid   (b) iron
   (c) folic acid          (d) ascorbic acid

6. Bilirubin is normally derived from
   (a) liver         (b) old red blood cells
   (c) gall bladder  (d) jaundice

7. Transfused blood which has been properly cross-matched against the patient's blood is unlikely to cause
   (a) rigors   (b) an allergic reaction
   (c) transmission of infection
   (d) an incompatible blood group reaction

8 Blood for transfusion is stored at

   (a) 0° C     (b) 3° C     (c) 4–6° C     (d) 10° C

9 Hypochromic anaemia may be due to deficiency of

   (a) thyroxine     (b) folic acid     (c) iron     (d) iodine

10 Anaemia due to iron deficiency is not caused by

   (a) dietary deficiency of iron     (b) chronic haemorrhage
   (c) disorders of intestinal absorption
   (d) haemolytic anaemia

11 Pernicious anaemia is vitamin B12 deficiency anaemia due to

   (a) gastrectomy     (b) dietary deficiency of vitamin B12
   (c) malabsorption due to intestinal disease
   (d) hereditary defect leading to atrophy of the gastric mucosa

12 The intrinsic factor is

   (a) hydrochloric acid
   (b) a protein secreted by gastric glands
   (c) a hormone secreted by gastric glands     (d) pepsin

13 The extrinsic factor is

   (a) hydrochloric acid     (b) vitamin B12
   (c) pepsin     (d) a hormone

14 In pernicious anaemia the system not involved is

   (a) digestive     (b) endocrine     (c) nervous     (d) blood

15 Pernicious anaemia is initiated by

   (a) anaemia     (b) vitamin B12 deficiency
   (c) an hereditary defect     (d) lack of intrinsic factor

16 Aplastic anaemia is due to

   (a) radiation or toxins damaging the bone marrow
   (b) vitamin C deficiency
   (c) hypersplenism     (d) folate deficiency

# Blood and Lymphoreticular System

17 Rupture of red blood cells by antibodies or toxins is called

   (a) haemolysis    (b) haemostasis
   (c) thrombolysis   (d) haemopoiesis

18 Polymorphonuclear leucocytes (polymorphs) are

   (a) non-phagocytic   (b) phagocytic
   (c) antibody-producing
   (d) phagocytic and antibody-producing

19 An increase in the number of normal white cells in the blood is called

   (a) leukaemia   (b) leucocytosis
   (c) leucopenia  (d) polychromasia

20 Which is the best answer? The presenting signs and symptoms of acute leukaemia are usually

   (a) fever, haemorrhages, sore throat, anaemia, leucocytosis
   (b) an increased number of white blood cells, usually in children
   (c) headache, drowsiness, and fits, due to leukaemic meningitis
   (d) enlarged lymph nodes and hepatomegaly

21 Acute leukaemia is treated with

   (a) radiotherapy   (b) prednisolone plus radiotherapy
   (c) vincristine
   (d) cytotoxic drugs, prednisolone and radiotherapy

22 A low platelet count is known as

   (a) thrombocytopenia   (b) thrombocythaemia
   (c) purpura   (d) ecchymoses

23 Normal lymph node function is to make lymphocytes and

   (a) filter off particles from the lymph
   (b) red blood cells
   (c) platelets   (d) to make lymph and destroy bacteria

24 Which of the following is not a function of the spleen?

   (a) to produce bilirubin  (b) to produce albumin
   (c) to produce lymphocytes
   (d) to destroy old red blood cells and platelets

25 Hodgkin's disease is primarily a

   (a) malignant disease of the blood  (b) type of leukaemia
   (c) benign growth of the lympho-reticular system
   (d) malignant growth of the lympho-reticular system

26 Cytotoxic (antineoplastic) drugs do not cause

   (a) depression of the bone marrow  (b) alopecia (baldness)
   (c) radiation sickness
   (d) ulceration of the mouth and intestines

# Answers

1 (d) (a), (b) and (c) are all functions of the plasma proteins. *Fluid leaves* the vascular system by means of the (hydrostatic) blood pressure, and *returns* by osmosis.
2 (c) The fluid portion of *clotted* blood is called *serum*.
3 (b) Immunoglobulins are antibodies.
4 (b) This question has been included as an example of the 'tricky' type sometimes asked. Only the marrow makes red *and* white cells. The spleen produces lymphocytes but not, in the normal adult, red blood cells.
5 (a) Ascorbic and folic acids and iron are required in red cell formation, deficiency leading to anaemia. Hydrochloric acid is unconnected with *marrow* function, although it helps to dissolve iron in the stomach and thus aid its absorption from the intestine.
6 (b) Bilirubin is *derived* from old red cells. It is *excreted* by the

# Blood and Lymphoreticular System

liver, *stored* in bile in the gall bladder. Jaundice is the *result* of either excessive bilirubin production, i.e. excessive breakdown of red cells (haemolytic anaemia), or failure of excretion of bilirubin which may be due to liver damage or to obstruction to bile flow.

7 (d) Cross-matching makes sure that the blood groups are compatible. It does not detect foreign materials in the plasma which may cause allergy, or infections such as malaria and hepatitis, which may be transmitted. Rigors may be due to a transfusion being given too rapidly, or to infection.

8 (c) Blood stores best at 4–6° C. Blood banks control the temperature within this range but ordinary refrigerators vary outside this range and should not be used for storing blood.

9 (c) Deficiency of thyroxine leads to normochromic anaemia. Deficiency of folic acid causes macrocytic anaemia. Iodine deficiency does not produce anaemia.

10 (d) Any haemorrhage leads to loss of iron but in chronic haemorrhage iron stores become depleted, then more iron may be lost than can be absorbed. In haemolytic anaemia the cells are destroyed in the body and the iron they contain is retained for further use.

11 (d) All four conditions may give rise to macrocytic anaemia due to lack of vitamin B12. Intrinsic factor is deficient (and, therefore, vitamin B12 cannot be absorbed), both after gastrectomy and in pernicious anaemia, but only the *hereditary* deficiency of intrinsic factor (due to gastric mucosal atrophy), is called pernicious anaemia.

12 (b) The gastric mucosa secretes hydrochloric acid, pepsin, and intrinsic factor (a protein, probably an enzyme), into the gastric lumen. Hormones are secreted directly into the blood.

13 (b) It requires the intrinsic factor for its absorption.

14 (b) The endocrine system is not involved in pernicious anaemia. The systems involved are the digestive (intrinsic factor deficiency), nervous (neuropathy), and blood (anaemia).

15 (c) This type of difficult question is sometimes asked. It can be understood by the following sequence:

1, An hereditary defect leads to 2, auto-immune damage to the stomach, which is followed by 3, lack of intrinsic factor, leading to 4, inability to absorb vitamin B12, hence 5, vitamin B12 deficiency resulting in 6, anaemia.

The *condition*, pernicious anaemia, is *initiated* by 1, but the *anaemia* itself is *due* to 5.

16 (a) X-rays, chloramphenicol, gold salts, and certain insecticides are well-known causes of damage to the bone marrow. (b), (c) and (d) may all cause anaemia (of different types), but not by damaging the marrow.
17 (a) Haemostasis is the checking of haemorrhage. Thrombolysis is the dissolving of clot. Haemopoiesis is the formation of blood.
18 (b) Polymorphs do not produce antibodies. For choice (d) to be correct, polymorphs would have to be *both* phagocytic *and* antibody-producing.
19 (b) In leukaemia the cells are *ab*normal. Leucopenia is a low white cell count. Polychromasia means 'several colours' and in haematology refers to stained red blood cells.
20 (a) These signs are present in most cases. Choice (b) has many causes, (c) and (d) are less common *presenting* signs.
21 (d) The other three choices are partly correct, but (d) is the best of the four answers.
22 (a) Thrombocythaemia is an *increased* platelet count. Purpura and ecchymoses may result *from* a low platelet count.
23 (a) Lymph is fluid returning from the tissues along the lymphatics. It is filtered, but not made, by the lymph nodes. Lymph nodes filter off particles, including bacteria. They help to destroy bacteria. Red blood cells and platelets are made by the bone marrow.
24 (b) The spleen filters off abnormal particles. It destroys old platelets and old red blood cells, haem from haemoglobin being made into bilirubin. The spleen produces lymphocytes but albumin is made by the liver.
25 (d) Hodgkin's disease is primarily a malignant growth of lymph nodes and spleen, not of the blood.
26 (c) Cytotoxic drugs may cause vomiting, but not *radiation* sickness.
   (a), (b) and (c) are common side-effects.

# 6 Cardiovascular System

1 In which order does the blood pass through the valves of the heart after it has entered the right atrium?

   (a) tricuspid, pulmonary, mitral, aortic
   (b) mitral, pulmonary, tricuspid, aortic
   (c) pulmonary, tricuspid, mitral, aortic
   (d) aortic, mitral, pulmonary, tricuspid

2 The sino-atrial node, regulated by the autonomic nervous system, sends out the following number of impulses each minute, approximately

   (a) 60   (b) 72   (c) 80 to 90   (d) 60 to 150

3 The 3 layers of an artery are

   (a) intima, endothelium, muscle
   (b) endothelium, muscle, elastic tissue
   (c) endothelium, muscle, media
   (d) intima, media, adventitia

4 Valves are present in

   (a) veins   (b) arteries   (c) arterioles   (d) capillaries

5 The following blood vessel(s) return blood to the heart

   (a) pulmonary arteries   (b) pulmonary veins
   (c) portal vein          (d) aorta

6 In atrial fibrillation the primary feature of the arterial pulse is that it is

   (a) slow   (b) rapid   (c) irregular   (d) regular

7 In atrial fibrillation the following should be recorded

   (a) the pulse at the left wrist
   (b) the pulse at the right wrist
   (c) the rate at the apex of the heart   (d) the carotid pulse

8 Blood pressure depends on

   (a) cardiac output         (b) blood volume
   (c) peripheral resistance   (d) all of them

9 An abnormally high blood pressure may be found because

   (a) the patient's arm is fat   (b) the patient is anxious
   (c) renal disease is present  (d) all of them

10 Systemic arterial hypertension may produce

   (a) left ventricular failure, cerebral haemorrhage, encephalopathy
   (b) pulmonary embolism    (c) cerebral embolism
   (d) portal hypertension and oesophageal varices

11 Shock should be treated by

   (a) leaving the patient as he is
   (b) warming the patient with hot-water bottles
   (c) removal of the cause, if possible
   (d) elevating the head of the bed

12 A patient is bleeding from an external wound. The most important initial treatment is

   (a) reassurance   (b) local pressure to stop the bleeding
   (c) oxygen        (d) blood transfusion

13 Breathlessness on lying down, relieved by sitting up is called

   (a) dyspnoea   (b) orthopnoea
   (c) hypopnoea  (d) hyperpnoea

14 In which of the following is digoxin not used?

   (a) bradycardia   (b) cardiac failure
   (c) atrial flutter   (d) rapid atrial fibrillation

15 During therapy with digoxin the heart rate per minute is kept between

   (a) 90 and 100  (b) 80 and 90
   (c) 60 and 80   (d) just below 60

# Cardiovascular System

16 Diuretics are used in order to

   (a) lower the plasma potassium level
   (b) raise the blood pressure
   (c) remove excessive fluid from the tissue
   (d) all of them

17 Which of the following is used as an analgesic and sedative?

   (a) aspirin      (b) phenylbutazone
   (c) morphine    (d) phenobarbitone

18 Ischaemic heart disease, chronic lung disease, and hyperthyroidism may all cause

   (a) anaemia           (b) cardiac failure
   (c) bacterial endocarditis  (d) cor pulmonale

19 Dyspnoea, cyanosis, distended jugular veins, and oedema of the legs are all signs of

   (a) chronic bronchitis
   (b) uncomplicated deep venous thrombosis
   (c) left ventricular failure    (d) congestive cardiac failure

20 In a patient with congestive cardiac failure the following should be observed

   (a) the present symptoms and signs and any changes in them
   (b) the appearance of new symptoms and signs
   (c) pulse (or apex) rate, rhythm and volume, temperature, respiratory rate and volume, and fluid intake and output
   (d) all of them

21 In congestive cardiac failure the usual salt content of the daily diet should be

   (a) nil (salt-free)   (b) low (3 g)
   (c) normal (10 g)   (d) high

22 A common complication of rheumatic mitral stenosis is

   (a) atrial fibrillation     (b) rheumatic fever
   (c) rheumatoid arthritis  (d) hypertension

23 'Cardiac asthma' (paroxysmal nocturnal dyspnoea) is due to

   (a) allergy
   (b) emphysema
   (c) ankle oedema
   (d) left ventricular failure

24 In acute pulmonary oedema the patient should

   (a) lie down
   (b) sit up with the legs raised
   (c) sit up with the legs hanging down
   (d) lie on the left side

25 Ischaemic coronary arterial disease is usually due to

   (a) arteriosclerosis
   (b) atheroma, with or without sclerosis
   (c) aneurysm
   (d) pain

26 Ischaemic heart disease does not cause

   (a) angina of effort
   (b) myocardial infarction
   (c) cardiac failure
   (d) coronary atheroma

27 Heredity, cigarette smoking, hypertension, and a high blood cholesterol predispose to

   (a) carcinoma of the bronchus
   (b) atheroma
   (c) chronic bronchitis
   (d) mitral stenosis

28 An attack of angina pectoris is treated with

   (a) rest in bed
   (b) trinitrin
   (c) anticoagulants
   (d) vitamin K

29 The management of a patient with angina does not include

   (a) increased animal (saturated) fat in the diet
   (b) reduction of weight if obese
   (c) giving up smoking
   (d) treatment of hypertension, if present

30 The symptoms of ischaemic heart disease are caused by a decrease of blood flowing

   (a) through the aortic valve
   (b) through the pulmonary artery
   (c) through the coronary arteries
   (d) to the heart muscle

# Cardiovascular System

31 The pain of coronary thrombosis differs from that of angina pectoris because it

(a) may come on at rest
(b) always comes on during exertion
(c) radiates down both arms
(d) lasts for a shorter period of time

32 In uncomplicated myocardial infarction, pyrexia, leucocytosis, and raised erythrocyte sedimentation rate (ESR), are due to

(a) infection  (b) products released from the dead tissue
(c) pulmonary embolism
(d) anxiety

33 Of the following, the commonest cause of heart disease is

(a) mitral stenosis  (b) diabetes mellitus
(c) hypertension  (d) endocarditis

34 In uncomplicated myocardial infarction, the early treatment is

(a) morphine, anticoagulants and diuretic
(b) morphine, rest, no smoking
(c) anticoagulants, diuretic, diet
(d) morphine, diuretic, procainamide

35 The first treatment of sudden loss of consciousness, absent carotid pulse, dilated pupils, and cessation of respiration, is

(a) cardiac massage and mouth-to-mouth respiration
(b) lignocaine
(c) oxygen and an intravenous drip containing sodium bicarbonate
(d) adrenaline, lignocaine and oxygen

36 Congenital heart disease is

(a) produced at birth  (b) present at birth
(c) produced in infancy  (d) disappears at birth

37 The treatment of infective (bacterial) endocarditis is

   (a) immediate high-dosage antibiotic
   (b) high doses of antibiotic after blood cultures have been taken, waiting two to three days, if necessary, before giving antibiotic.
   (c) low-dosage antibiotic immediately
   (d) immediate antibiotic followed by blood cultures for three to six days

38 Pericarditis is inflammation of the

   (a) lining of the valves of the heart    (b) pleura
   (c) outer covering of the heart
   (d) outer layer of the cardiac end of the stomach

39 Pulmonary emboli do not arise from the

   (a) right side of the heart    (b) veins in the legs
   (c) left side of the heart     (d) veins in the pelvis

40 The treatment for uncomplicated pulmonary embolism is

   (a) The patient should be nursed lying down, and given oxygen, morphine, anticoagulants
   (b) The patient should be nursed lying down and given oxygen, but no morphine since it depresses respiration
   (c) Anticoagulants    (d) both (b) and (c)

41 Atheroma (atherosclerosis) is

   (a) uniform deposition of fat in the intima of arteries
   (b) patchy deposition of fat in the intima of arteries
   (c) patchy deposition of fat in the intima of veins
   (d) uniform thickening of the intima and media by fibrosis (sclerosis)

42 Arterial obstruction in the leg is never due to

   (a) embolism    (b) phlebothrombosis
   (c) atheroma    (d) thrombosed aneurysm

# Cardiovascular System

43 Deep venous thrombosis is often prevented by

    (a) dehydration     (b) immobilisation
    (c) mobilisation     (d) operation

44 Following heart surgery all patients will need

    (a) digoxin     (b) oxygen
    (c) diuretic     (d) abundant i.v. fluid

45 One of the following is not a treatment for varicose veins

    (a) injection of sclerosant     (b) elastic stockings
    (c) surgical ligation     (d) anticoagulants

46 When measuring the blood pressure using a stethoscope, the diastolic pressure is recorded when the first sound

    (a) is heard     (b) becomes muffled     (c) disappears
    (d) both muffling and disappearance of the sound should be recorded

# Answers

1 (a)
2 (d) The *isolated* sino-atrial node sends out 60 impulses a minute, but when under autonomic nervous control (as specified in the question), it adjusts the rate according to the needs of the body.
3 (d) The intima consists of endothelial cells, the media of muscle and elastic tissue, and the adventitia (the outer layer) of fibrous tissue.
4 (a)
5 (b) The pulmonary veins convey blood from the lungs to the heart and are the only veins containing oxygenated blood.

6 (c) The pulse rate is usually rapid, sometimes slow, but *always* irregular.
7 (c) In atrial fibrillation some of the heart beats may not be felt at the wrist, resulting in a falsely low recording. Both weak and strong beats will be heard over the heart. It would be more informative to record both the apex rate *and* the pulse rate at the wrist, any difference is called the 'pulse deficit', but the question did not include this possibility.
8 (d) is the best answer. It may seem unfair, but a mark will be lost if (a), (b) or (c) has been chosen.
9 (d) See answer 8, above.
10 (a)
11 (c) A shocked patient requires treatment. The *food*-end of the bed may be elevated, not the head. Even moderate heat may burn a shocked patient since the skin is vasoconstricted and has a poor blood flow, hence heat remains localised and is not carried away to be redistributed ('diluted') throughout the body.
12 (b) Reassurance is part of the treatment but it is *more important* to control haemorrhage. Blood transfusion is not part of the *initial* treatment since it takes time to determine the patient's blood group and perform a cross-matching. Transfusion may not be needed if blood loss is less than 1 l.
13 (b) 'Orthopnoea' specifically refers to breathlessness relieved by sitting up and is therefore the best answer, and although it is true that 'dyspnoea' refers to *any* form of breathlessness a mark is lost if 'dyspnoea' is chosen.
14 (a) Digoxin slows the heart rate and is likely to worsen bradycardia.
15 (c) The heart rate is usually kept near 70, but sometimes the clinical response is inadequate at this dosage of digoxin and a larger dose, slowing the heart rate below 70, may be required.
16 (c) Diuretics may lead to hypokalaemia but this is a side-effect. They are often used in order to *lower* the blood pressure in hypertension.
17 (c) Aspirin and phenylbutazone are not sedatives, phenobarbitone is not an analgesic.
18 (b) Cor pulmonale is heart failure due to lung disease only.
19 (d) In chronic bronchitis and in left ventricular failure the jugular veins are not distended (except during coughing), and there is no peripheral oedema. Dyspnoea, cyanosis and dis-

tended jugular veins do not occur in *uncomplicated* deep venous thrombosis.
20 (d)
21 (b) By not adding salt at the table or in the cooking, intake is reduced to about 3 g daily, the *usual* amount allowed in cardiac failure. A salt-free diet would be better but, since most food contains some salt, such a diet is difficult to prepare and is only used in cases resisting other forms of treatment.
22 (a) Rheumatic fever is a *cause*, not a complication, of mitral stenosis.
23 (d) In 'cardiac asthma', failure of the left ventricle to pump out the blood it receives from the lungs produces pulmonary congestion with an increased pressure in the pulmonary capillaries, leading to escape of fluid from the capillaries into the pulmonary interstitial tissue, and (when the capacity of the lymphatics is exceeded), into the alveoli (pulmonary oedema), hence a feeling of suffocation and tightness in the chest.
Allergy may cause *bronchial* asthma.
24 (c) Sitting up with the legs hanging down helps to reduce the venous return to the heart and reduces the pulmonary oedema. Lying down would produce more severe dyspnoea, as might raising the legs.
25 (b) This question has been set, not as a catch question, but to make sure that the difference between atheroma and arteriosclerosis is understood, since this type of awkward question is sometimes encountered in examinations. Arteriosclerosis is *any* form of sclerosis (hardening) of arteries and has several causes, only one of which is atherosclerosis. Atheroma (with or without sclerosis) is usually the cause of ischaemic coronary arterial disease and is, therefore, the better answer. The other forms of arteriosclerosis either do not cause ischaemia or rarely do so.
26 (d) Ischaemic heart disease *does* cause (a), (b), and (c) and it is a *result* not a *cause* of coronary atheroma.
27 (b) Hypertension and hypercholesterolaemia do not predispose to (a), (c), or (d).
28 (b) Rest *in bed* is not necessary in ordinary angina. Anticoagulants are ineffective. Vitamin K is irrelevant.
29 (a) A *reduction* in the intake of saturated fat is desirable.
30 (d) *Symptoms* are due to ischaemia of heart muscle.
31 (a) Both may follow exertion but they *differ* in that the pain

of myocardial infarction often comes on at rest, whereas angina rarely does so. The pain may radiate down one or both arms both in angina and in myocardial infarction. The pain of infarction lasts longer (hours) than that of angina (minutes).

32 (b) In *un*complicated infarction there is no pulmonary embolism or infection.
Anxiety does not produce a leucocytosis or raise the ESR.

33 (c)

34 (b) Morphine, rest and prohibition of smoking are *all* correct therapy (smoking predisposes to arrhythmias, which may be fatal).
A diuretic is not necessary in *un*complicated infarction, therefore, (a), (c) and (d) are incorrect even though procainamide may be used prophylactically to prevent arrhythmia. Diet is not an *immediate* treatment. Anticoagulants do not affect coronary atheroma and do not improve the prognosis in myocardial infarction, but may be used to prevent thromboembolism.

35 (a) The condition described is cardiac arrest. The *first* treatment is resuscitation, the other choices, (b), (c), and (d), may also be necessary, but *after* resuscitation has been started.

36 (b) 'Congenital' means present at birth. Congenital heart disease occurs in the fetus, usually in the first 3 months of pregnancy.

37 (b) Immediate antibiotic prevents the growth of organisms in culture.
If the organism cannot be grown, its sensitivity to antibiotic (which is essential to know in endocarditis) cannot be tested.

38 (c) The others are endocarditis (a), pleurisy (b), and peritonitis (d).

39 (c) Any emboli arising from a blood clot in the left side of the heart enter the aorta and impact in the systemic arterial circulation e.g. renal artery. Emboli from veins in the legs or pelvis pass along the inferior vena cava into the right side of the heart; these, or emboli from the right side of the heart then travel into the pulmonary artery, forming pulmonary emboli.

40 (a) The patient is nursed flat, since shock is usually present.
The degree of respiratory depression produced by morphine is not of significance in *uncomplicated* pulmonary embolism

# Cardiovascular System

and its benefits (relief of anxiety, sedation, analgesia, and help in reducing shock) outweigh its disadvantages.

If pulmonary embolism was complicated by the patient having chronic bronchitis and emphysema, morphine might not be given.

41 (b) Atheroma is patchy and does not affect veins.
42 (b) Phlebothrombosis is thrombosis of veins, not arteries.
43 (c) Dehydration, immobilisation, and operation predispose to venous thrombosis.
44 (b) Digoxin is not required unless there is tachycardia or atrial fibrillation.
A diuretic is needed only if cardiac failure ensues.
Intravenous fluid is given with caution so as not to overload the circulation.
45 (d)
46 You may have a mark for (b), (c), or (d) but lose one for (a).
This question has been included so as to point out that there is still a controversy as to whether (b) or (c) shoudl be recorded as the diastolic pressure. A recent suggestion is that both muffling and disappearance of the sound should be recorded, e.g. 120/80–60.

# 7 The Respiratory System

1 The function of the nasal mucosa is to
   (a) moisten and warm the air and trap particles
   (b) trap particles and move mucus into the larynx
   (c) trap particles, move mucus into the larynx, and absorb oxygen
   (d) trap particles, absorb oxygen, and provide the sense of smell

2 The function of the Eustachian tube is to
   (a) allow secretions from the external auditory meatus to drain into the pharynx
   (b) allow the auditory ossicles free movement
   (c) protect the inner ear
   (d) keep the air pressure the same on each side of the tympanic membrane

3 Gaseous exchange in the lungs takes place across the walls of the
   (a) trachea   (b) bronchi   (c) alveoli   (d) bronchioles

4 How many layers is the pleura composed of?
   (a) one   (b) two   (c) three   (d) four

5 The normal pleural cavity contains
   (a) oxygen and carbon dioxide   (b) oxygen
   (c) 350 ml of fluid   (d) a thin film of fluid

6 The normal respiratory rate per minute at rest is approximately
   (a) 20   (b) 18   (c) 14   (d) 10

Respiratory System

7 When the diaphragm relaxes it moves upwards because of

  (a) contraction of the abdominal muscles
  (b) expansion of the chest
  (c) contraction of the diaphragm
  (d) the elastic recoil of the lungs

8 Hypoxaemia is a low

  (a) oxalate in the blood    (b) oxygen level in the lungs
  (c) oxygen level in the air
  (d) oxygen level in the arterial blood

9 The coughing up of blood is called

  (a) haemoptysis    (b) haematemesis
  (c) melaena        (d) haemolytic

10 Sputum consists of

  (a) saliva    (b) secretions of the respiratory tract only
  (c) secretions of the respiratory tract and inhaled particles
  (d) saliva plus respiratory tract secretions and inhaled particles

11 Bronchodilators relieve bronchial narrowing by

  (a) relaxing smooth muscle
  (b) reducing oedema of the mucosa
  (c) dilating the bronchial blood vessels
  (d) reducing inflammation

12 Adrenaline does not

  (a) constrict bronchi    (b) dilate bronchi
  (c) increase the heart rate
  (d) relax the bladder detrusor muscle

13 The amount of oxygen given to a patient with chronic bronchitis and emphysema is

  (a) 28%    (b) 40%    (c) 78%    (d) 6 to 10 litres/minute

14 A patient, with tracheostomy tubes correctly in place, has noisy breathing and is restless. Attention is therefore required

   (a) to the outer tube   (b) to the inner tube
   (c) to the tracheobronchial airway
   (d) attention is not required

15 The immediate treatment for epistaxis (nose bleeding) is

   (a) tilting the head backwards
   (b) lowering the head forwards
   (c) squeezing the nostrils for several minutes
   (d) blood transfusion

16 Which of the following does not complicate tonsillitis?

   (a) otitis media and quinsy   (b) acute rheumatic fever
   (c) acute glomerulonephritis   (d) acute pyelonephritis

17 Chronic bronchitis is commonly due to

   (a) pneumonia   (b) tobacco smoke
   (c) pneumothorax   (d) humid air

18 Overdistension of alveoli is called

   (a) empyema   (b) emphysema
   (c) pneumothorax   (d) alveolitis

19 Pulmonary emphysema is not caused by

   (a) chronic bronchitis   (b) right-sided heart failure
   (c) smoking   (d) pneumoconiosis

20 Which one of the following is not a cause of asthma?

   (a) infection of bronchi   (b) overactive sympathetic nerves
   (c) allergy   (d) overactive vagus nerves

21 An acute attack of asthma is treated with

   (a) 60% oxygen, sympathomimetics and antihistamine
   (b) 30% oxygen, isoprenaline and antihistamine
   (c) 28% oxygen, disodium cromoglycate and salbutamol
   (d) 60% oxygen and sympathomimetics

# Respiratory System

22 Which of the following is not used in bacterial pneumonia?

   (a) oxygen  (b) tetracycline
   (c) semi-solid diet  (d) diuretic

23 A lung abscess is least likely to be due to

   (a) asthma  (b) pneumonia
   (c) bronchial carcinoma  (d) tuberculosis

24 In bronchiectasis there is

   (a) displacement of the bronchi
   (b) constriction of bronchi
   (c) dilatation of bronchi
   (d) constriction of bronchioles

25 Of the following, the most important treatment for infected bronchiectasis is

   (a) humidified air  (b) penicillin
   (c) postural drainage  (b) abundant fluids

26 Pneumoconiosis may be due to the inhalation of

   (a) pollen  (b) pigeon or parrot droppings
   (c) dust from mouldy hay  (d) silica and coal dust

27 Most cases of carcinoma of the bronchus are due to

   (a) inhaling asbestos particles  (b) smoking cigarettes
   (c) working where there are chromium or nickel fumes
   (d) repeatedly being in a room full of cigarette smoke

28 What percentage of malignant disease in males is due to carcinoma of the bronchus?

   (a) 12%  (b) 24%  (c) 40%  (d) 8%

29 Fibrocystic disease (mucoviscidosis) is due to

   (a) steatorrhoea  (b) a genetic defect
   (c) viscid mucus  (d) repeated pneumonitis

30 Air in the pleural cavity is called

   (a) pneumothorax    (b) atelectasis
   (c) hydrothorax     (d) pleurisy

31 Which of the following is not a complication of a fractured rib?

   (a) haemothorax     (b) pulmonary emphysema
   (c) pneumothorax    (d) surgical emphysema

32 After lobectomy the nursing care should be concentrated on

   (a) antibiotic therapy  (b) fluid balance
   (c) bronchodilators     (d) making the patient cough

33 In respiratory failure the first treatment is

   (a) artificial respiration  (b) tracheostomy
   (c) ensure a clear airway   (d) oxygen

## Answers

1 (a) Its cilia move mucus into the *pharynx*, not into the larynx. It does not absorb any appreciable amount of oxygen, hence (c) and (d) are wrong despite the fact that they contain *some* correct functions.
2 (d) Secretions (wax) drain *externally* to the auricle, the inner end being closed by the tympanic membrane.
3 (c)
4 (b) The visceral pleura lining the lungs and the parietal pleura lining the thoracic wall and upper surface of the diaphragm.
5 (d) A thin layer of lubricating fluid secreted by the pleural cells.
6 (c) The normal range is 12 to 16, average 14.

# Respiratory System

7  (d) This is aided by the higher intra-abdominal pressure.
8  (d)
9  (a) Haematemesis is the vomiting of blood, melaena refers to black faeces due to blood, and haemolytic means blood 'dissolving', i.e. rupture of red blood cells.
10 (c) Saliva is not sputum, even when mixed with it.
11 (a) Corticosteroids may reduce inflammation and oedema, but are not primarily bronchodilators.
12 (a) It is correct to state that adrenaline does *not* constrict bronchi.
13 (a) Concentrations higher than 35% may lead to carbon dioxide narcosis in patients with chronic bronchitis and emphysema.
14 (c) Tracheobronchial suction, at least, is likely to be required. The question states that the tracheostomy tubes themselves are *not* displaced.
15 (c) Bleeding is usually from a small area near the front of the nose and is prevented by local pressure. Tilting the head merely allows the blood to flow out of the nostril, or down the throat! Blood transfusion may or may not be required, but is not *immediate* treatment.
16 (d) All the others may complicate tonsillitis.
17 (b) Pneumonia or pneumothorax may be predisposed by chronic bronchitis, not vice versa.
18 (b) Empyema is a collection of pus. Pneumothorax is air in the pleural 'cavity'. Alveolitis is *inflammation* of the alveoli.
19 (b)
20 (b) Increased activity of sympathetic nerves *dilates* bronchi, the other choices may all produce asthma and bronchoconstriction.
21 (d) 60% oxygen should be given in asthma, and, to dilate the bronchi, sympathomimetics. Antihistamines dry the secretions, which is undesirable, and are ineffective. Disodium cromoglycate acts if taken prophylactically, but not once an acute attack is in progress.
22 (d) Fluid intake should be high. Diuretics are unnecessary and are contraindicated.
23 (a)
24 (c)
25 (c) Usually, in bronchiectasis, infection is due to several organisms which are often resistant to penicillin. Patients are not unduly prone to dehydration.

26 (d) Pneumoconioses are due to *mineral* dusts. (a), (b) and (c) are not minerals. Pollen allergy may affect the nose (hay fever) or bronchi (asthma), and bird droppings and mouldy hay may cause allergic alveolitis, but they do *not* cause pneumoconiosis.
27 (b) Carcinoma of the bronchus is usually due to cigarette smoking. Occasional cases are due to chromium or nickel fumes or asbestos particles.
Choice (d) is unproven.
28 (c)
29 (b) An autosomal recessive genetic defect leading to viscid secretions.
Choices (a), (c) and (d) *result from* the disease.
30 (a) Atelectasis = unexpanded lung, hydrothorax = pleural effusion, pleurisy = pleural inflammation.
31 (b) Pulmonary emphysema is distension of the air sacs, associated with e.g. chronic bronchitis. This must not be confused with surgical emphysema in which air enters the tissues from the lungs, usually through an injury to the lung.
32 (d) Every hour the wound should be supported and the patient encouraged to cough. Bronchodilators are seldom required, fluid balance is rarely a problem, and antibiotic therapy cannot be described as concentrated nursing care.
33 (c) Neither artificial respiration nor oxygen are of use if the airway is obstructed.

# 8 The Digestive System

## PART 1

1 Digestion of food begins in the
   - (a) mouth
   - (b) oesophagus
   - (c) stomach
   - (d) intestine

2 Proteins primarily consist of
   - (a) sugars
   - (b) amino acids
   - (c) starches
   - (d) triglycerides

3 For their absorption vitamins A, D, E and K require
   - (a) gastric juice
   - (b) trypsin
   - (c) bile
   - (d) amylase

4 Thrush (*Candida*, Monilia) infection is treated with
   - (a) penicillin
   - (b) tetracycline
   - (c) cortisone
   - (d) nystatin

5 The number of teeth in the adult is
   - (a) 32
   - (b) 30
   - (c) 28
   - (d) 20

6 One of the following is not a cause of dysphagia
   - (a) stomatitis
   - (b) glossitis
   - (c) multiple sclerosis
   - (d) pharyngitis

7 In carcinoma of the oesophagus
   - (a) dysphagia is not a problem
   - (b) digested food regurgitates
   - (c) undigested food regurgitates
   - (d) vomiting predominates

8 Hiatus hernia is

   (a) failure of relaxation of the oesophagus
   (b) protrusion of part of the stomach into the chest
   (c) failure of relaxation of the cardiac end of the stomach
   (d) protrusion of the lower end of the oesophagus into the abdomen

9 Reflux oesophagitis is treated with

   (a) weight reduction, small meals, avoidance of stooping
   (b) antacids
   (c) gastrectomy and (a)    (d) both (a) and (b)

10 The upper part of the stomach normally

   (a) is empty         (b) secretes trypsin
   (c) contains fluid   (d) contains air

11 How many of the following are functions of the stomach? Secretion of hydrochloric acid, mucus, enzymes and a hormone, and to mix food

   (a) two    (b) three    (c) four    (d) all of them

12 Gastric secretion and motility are controlled by

   (a) vagus nerves only    (b) vagus nerves and gastrin
   (c) gastrin only         (d) sympathetic nerves

13 Vomiting may be due to disease of the

   (a) abdomen, nervous system, labyrinth, kidney
   (b) eye, kidney
   (c) both (a) and (b)    (d) (a), (b) and the endocrine system

14 An absence of hydrochloric acid secretion by the stomach is

   (a) anorexia      (b) nausea
   (c) achlorhydria  (d) gastritis

15 Antispasmodic drugs are

   (a) anticholinergic            (b) vagus nerve stimulants
   (c) sympathetic stimulants     (d) sympathetic depressants

# Digestive System

16 Peptic ulceration is due to the action of
   (a) pepsin alone  (b) pepsin and hydrochloric acid
   (c) mucus  (d) antacid

17 Perforation of a peptic ulcer leads to
   (a) severe haemorrhage  (b) pyloric stenosis
   (c) oedema of the legs
   (d) release of the gastric contents into the peritoneal cavity

18 The test performed for suspected slight bleeding from a peptic ulcer is
   (a) blood count for anaemia  (b) faeces for occult blood
   (c) barium meal
   (d) examine faeces for bright red blood

19 The treatment of an uncomplicated peptic ulcer is usually
   (a) medical  (b) surgical
   (c) radiotherapy  (d) cytotoxic drugs

20 Which of the following is the most important treatment in duodenal ulcer?
   (a) milk and antacid
   (b) vitamins, properly chewed food and milk
   (c) fish and milk  (d) antacid, rest and regular meals

21 Vomit containing dark brown granular material ('coffee-grounds') indicates
   (a) peptic ulcer  (b) that blood has been in the stomach
   (c) that bleeding is occurring in the stomach
   (d) carcinoma of the stomach

22 Treatment of haematemesis always includes
   (a) treatment of shock  (b) blood transfusion
   (c) gastrectomy  (d) desmopressin

23 The vomiting of food taken the previous day indicates
   (a) gastric ulcer  (b) pyloric obstruction
   (c) duodenal ulcer  (d) carcinoma of the stomach

24 Pyloric stenosis may be due to

(a) a congenital cause in infants  (b) blood disease
(c) hiatus hernia
(d) peptic ulceration of the cardiac end of the stomach

25 The treatment of pyloric stenosis is usually

(a) as for peptic ulcer  (b) immediate partial gastrectomy
(c) fluid diet and vitamins
(d) rehydration, protein and vitamins followed by operation

26 Which is the best description of the symptoms and signs of carcinoma of the stomach?

(a) anaemia, tiredness, pallor, smooth tongue
(b) nausea, vomiting, fullness after large meals, abdominal pain
(c) anaemia, anorexia, vomiting, weight loss, mass in epigastrium
(d) tiredness, pallor, smooth tongue, anorexia, weight loss

27 When a peptic ulcer perforates the pain is

(a) severe and colicky  (b) moderate and burning
(c) sudden and severe  (d) slight

28 Vagotomy is performed in order to

(a) decrease gastric motility
(b) decrease gastric acid secretion
(c) increase gastric acid secretion
(d) increase gastric motility and emptying rate

29 In the absence of wound haematoma or infection, pyrexia 48 hours after an operation may be due to

(a) any operation  (b) secondary haemorrhage
(c) deep venous thrombosis  (d) mild anaemia

# Digestive System

30  A surgical wound for a gastric operation consists of the incision in the
   (a) skin only    (b) skin and fascia only
   (c) skin, fascia and muscles
   (d) skin, fascia, muscles and all the deeper organs which have been opened

31  The aim of post-operative deep breathing exercises is to
   (a) increase the blood oxygen level
   (b) improve the oxygen supply to the brain
   (c) prevent pulmonary complications
   (d) eliminate anaesthetic gases

32  Peritonitis, bronchopneumonia, vomiting, or haemorrhage may all be likely complications of
   (a) gastrectomy    (b) pneumonectomy
   (c) herniorrhaphy    (d) amputation of a limb

33  The most important part of treatment for a perforated peptic ulcer is
   (a) rest in bed and fluid balance chart    (b) morphine
   (c) gastric aspiration, rehydration and antibiotic
   (d) abdominal X-ray

## PART 2

34  The pancreas is
   (a) an exocrine gland    (b) an endocrine gland
   (c) both    (d) neither

35  The secretion of pancreatic juice is stimulated by
   (a) the vagus nerve    (b) hormones
   (c) both    (d) neither

36 Which one of the following is not a cause of acute pancreatitis?

    (a) cholecystitis    (b) virus infection
    (c) alcoholism    (d) colitis

37 The best treatment for uncomplicated acute pancreatitis is

    (a) gastric aspiration and an intravenous drip
    (b) pethidine, antibiotic and an anticholinergic drug
    (c) (a) plus (b)    (d) surgery and (a) plus (b)

38 Pale bulky stools which float on water may be due to chronic

    (a) cholecystitis    (b) pancreatitis
    (c) colitis    (d) gastritis

39 Faeces may be pale and bulky and float on water because

    (a) the diet contains 50% more fat than normal
    (b) of an excess of carbohydrate in the diet, which is changed to fat
    (c) of gastritis    (d) there is failure to absorb fat

40 Carcinoma of the pancreas may cause jaundice due to

    (a) obstruction of the common bile duct    (b) pancreatitis
    (c) obstruction of the cystic bile duct
    (d) lymphatic obstruction

41 In mucoviscidosis (fibrocystic disease) the treatment is

    (a) pancreatic extract    (b) high salt diet
    (c) low carbohydrate diet    (d) high fat diet

42 The absorptive surface area of the intestinal mucosa is increased by

    (a) folds in the muscular layer    (b) villi
    (c) lacteals    (d) goblet cells

43 Regurgitation of intestinal contents into the small intestine is prevented by the

    (a) pyloric sphincter    (b) ileocaecal valve
    (c) mitral valve    (d) anal sphincter

# Digestive System

44 The pancreatic and bile ducts enter the

   (a) pylorus   (b) duodenum   (c) jejunum   (d) ileum

45 The small intestinal mucosa does not provide the function of

   (a) absorption   (b) protection
   (c) secretion   (d) peristalsis

46 Emulsification of fat in the duodenum is achieved by the action of

   (a) bile pigments   (b) lipase
   (c) chyme   (d) bile salts

47 Colicky abdominal pain is due to

   (a) peptic ulcer   (b) peritonitis
   (c) smooth muscle spasm   (d) paralytic ileus

48 Crohn's disease, intussusception, strangulated hernia and adhesions may all directly cause

   (a) mesenteric thrombosis   (b) Meckel's diverticulum
   (c) intestinal obstruction   (d) peritonitis

49 Colic, mucocele, jaundice or pancreatitis may all complicate

   (a) kidney stones   (b) gall stones
   (c) intestinal obstruction   (d) alcoholism

50 The symptoms of diagnostic importance in mechanical intestinal obstruction are

   (a) vomiting, colic, constipation
   (b) abdominal distension, concentrated urine
   (c) vomiting, burning pain, diarrhoea, dehydration
   (d) colicky pain, dehydration, dry tongue, diarrhoea

51 The treatment of intestinal obstruction is

   (a) observation for 24 hours, gastric aspiration and intravenous drip
   (b) always surgical
   (c) purgative and antibiotic
   (d) not necessarily any one of these

52 Before operation in acute intestinal obstruction the patient is given

 (a) an aperient  (b) an intravenous infusion
 (c) fluid by mouth  (d) blood transfusion

53 The presence of excess fat in the stools is called

 (a) enteropathy  (b) diarrhoea
 (c) steatorrhoea  (d) sprue

54 Coeliac disease is treated with a diet containing

 (a) gluten  (b) wheat or rye
 (c) no fat  (d) no wheat or rye

55 In Crohn's disease the wall of the terminal ileum is

 (a) thinned  (b) thickened  (c) dilated  (d) neoplastic

56 Crohn's disease is due to

 (a) inflammation  (b) tumour
 (c) trauma  (d) atheroma

57 Food poisoning is not due to

 (a) allergy to food  (b) bacteria
 (c) bacterial toxins  (d) chemical poisons in food

58 The caecum is part of the

 (a) ileum  (b) colon
 (c) rectum  (d) is a separate organ

59 The appendix opens from the

 (a) ileum  (b) caecum  (c) colon  (d) rectum

60 Acute appendicitis usually begins with

 (a) pain in the right iliac fossa  (b) diarrhoea
 (c) pain in the right hypochondrium  (d) colicky pain

# Digestive System

61 The most satisfactory treatment for acute appendicitis is

   (a) early appendicectomy   (b) late appendicectomy
   (c) observation only   (d) medical treatment

62 The large intestine can absorb

   (a) water   (b) protein   (c) vitamin B12   (d) cellulose

63 A small amount of bright red blood in the faeces may be due to

   (a) gastric ulcer   (b) hiatus hernia
   (c) coeliac disease   (d) colitis

64 One of the following is not a cause of constipation

   (a) spastic colon   (b) anorexia
   (c) hyperthyroidism   (d) hypothyroidism

65 The treatment of acute abdominal pain

   (a) is immediate operation
   (b) always needs operation, but not always urgently
   (c) is always medical   (d) may be medical or surgical

66 Which of the following is not an early (within hours) post-operative complication?

   (a) paralytic ileus   (b) pulmonary collapse
   (c) intestinal obstruction from adhesions
   (d) haemorrhage

67 An ileostomy may be performed as part of the operation for

   (a) pyloric stenosis   (b) ulcerative colitis
   (c) rectal carcinoma
   (d) diverticulosis of the sigmoid colon

68 In acute ulcerative colitis the diet should be

   (a) high protein, low residue   (b) low protein, low residue
   (c) low calorie, high residue   (d) none of these

69 Long-term treatment of chronic diarrhoea in ulcerative colitis is with

   (a) codeine phosphate   (b) codeine compound
   (c) tincture of opium   (d) morphine

70 One of the following is not used in treating ulcerative colitis

   (a) fludrocortisone   (b) prednisolone
   (c) sulphasalazine    (d) hydrocortisone

71 A diverticulum of the colon is a

   (a) track joining two parts of the mucosa
   (b) pouch of mucosa
   (c) cyst in the muscle   (d) inflammation of the colon

72 Most attacks of diverticulitis are treated

   (a) with local surgery         (b) surgically plus antibiotic
   (c) by performing colectomy    (d) medically

73 A track joining two epithelial surfaces is called a

   (a) diverticulum   (b) stoma   (c) fistula   (d) fissure

74 Investigations for carcinoma of the large intestine may include

   (a) sigmoidoscopy and biopsy
   (b) blood count and faeces for occult blood
   (c) barium enema   (d) all of these

75 Before colectomy post-operative infection arising from cutting the bowel can be diminished by giving

   (a) oral penicillin and purgatives
   (b) evacuant enemata and oral neomycin
   (c) oral ampicillin and abundant fluid   (d) both (a) plus (c)

76 Haemorrhage and prolapse often complicate

   (a) appendicitis   (b) spastic colon
   (c) haemorrhoids   (d) peritonitis

# Digestive System

77 A common complication of peritonitis is

(a) haematemesis  (b) colic
(c) paralytic ileus  (d) diarrhoea

78 A hernia is the protrusion of a part of the body through

(a) a normal opening  (b) an abnormal opening
(c) any opening  (d) the skin

79 One of the following is not a serous membrane

(a) peritoneum  (b) synovium
(c) periosteum  (d) pericardium

# Answers

## PART 1

1 (a) Digestion begins with chewing and salivary amylase.
2 (b) Proteins consist of chains of amino acids. They *may* have other molecules *attached*, e.g. fat (producing lipoprotein) or sugar (forming glycoprotein).
3 (c) Vitamins A, D, E and K are fat soluble and, along with fat, require emulsification by bile salts for their absorption.
4 (d) Antibiotics such as tetracycline predispose to *Candida* infection by suppressing the normal flora and allowing fungal growth.
5 (a)
6 (a) The tongue and pharynx are involved in swallowing thus, if inflamed, may cause painful or difficult swallowing (dysphagia). Paralysis of the muscles used in swallowing, as may occur in multiple sclerosis, will cause difficulty in swallowing.
7 (c) The carcinoma obstructs the oesophagus, hence difficulty in swallowing and the collection of *un*digested food in the

oesophagus. This food regurgitates (*pseudo* vomiting), true vomiting being unusual.
8 (b) Failure of relaxation of the oesophagus is called achalasia.
9 (d) Various operations may be used, but gastrectomy is *not* one of them.
10 (d) It contains swallowed air.
11 (d)
12 (b)
13 (d) Vomiting may occur in glaucoma, renal colic, migraine, Addison's disease, diabetic ketosis and labyrinthitis, to mention only a few causes.
14 (c) 'a' = without, 'chlorhydria' = hydrochloric acid.
15 (a) Antispasmodic drugs (e.g. atropine) inhibit cholinergic action such as vagal nerve activity. They do not have any direct action on the sympathetic system.
16 (b) Gastric mucus and antacids *protect* against peptic ulceration.
17 (d) Perforation must not be confused with haemmorhage from an ulcer.
Perforation is due to ulceration of the peritoneum. Haemorrhage is due to ulceration of a blood vessel.
18 (b) *Slight* bleeding is not visible in the faeces but will give a positive test for occult blood. Larger amounts (above 100 ml) appear black or very dark brown owing to partial digestion in the gut. Anaemia may or may not be present if bleeding is slight and in any case may have other causes, e.g. a milk diet lacking in iron.
19 (a) Surgical treatment is more likely to be used for complications.
Radiotherapy and cytotoxins are contra-indicated.
20 (d) Antacid and rest is more important than any *specific* type of diet so long as irritant foods (e.g. spices, pickles, and chipped potatoes) are avoided and bland food is taken frequently. Milk is used for its convenience and because it has an antacid action, but a finely minced full diet is also suitable and contains a greater range of minerals and vitamins than does milk.
21 (b) 'Coffee-grounds' vomit indicates blood which has been altered by gastric juice. It does not necessarily mean that bleeding is taking place in the stomach since swallowed blood (e.g. from a bleeding nose) will also change its appearance after being in the stomach for a while.

# Digestive System

22 (a) Blood transfusion is not always required. Haematemesis has several causes thus gastrectomy or desmopressin may not be the appropriate treatment.

23 (b) It indicates pyloric obstruction from *any* cause, including carcinoma of the stomach, but it does not indicate carcinoma of the stomach *specifically*. The vomiting of food *taken the previous day* does not occur in gastric or duodenal ulcer uncomplicated by gastric stenosis.

24 (a) Congenital hypertrophic pyloric stenosis in infants is due to thickening (hypertrophy) of the pylorus. (c) and (d) refer to the upper (cardiac) end of the stomach, not the lower end (pylorus).

25 (d) The patient is usually dehydrated and has lost weight owing to vomiting. Operation is, therefore, performed after his condition has been improved.

26 (c) A mass in the epigastrium, if present, is particularly important. Choice (a) describes only anaemia. In carcinoma of the stomach fullness is felt after *small* meals, and there is often abdominal discomfort rather than distinct pain.

27 (c) The pain is sudden, severe and persistent.

28 (b) The aim of vagotomy is to decrease gastric acid secretion. As an *unwanted* effect it also decreases gastric motility.

29 (c) Pyrexia due to operative trauma seldom lasts longer than 24 hours. Secondary haemorrhage occurs at 7 to 10 (not two) days.

30 (d) 'A wound' includes all the tissues damaged or incised.

31 (c) In the absence of pulmonary complications deep breathing exercises do not increase the oxygen level of the blood or brain. Exercises should be continued for several days—long after anaesthetics have been eliminated.

32 (a) Peritonitis does not complicate (b) or (d) and although it is a possible complication of the repair of a hernia it is an *un*likely one.

33 (c) The other three choices although important are not the *most* important part of the treatment.

# PART 2

34 (c) The pancreas secretes enzymes into the gut from exocrine glands, and hormones into the blood from the islets of Langerhans (endocrine cells).

35 (c) The hormones are secretin and cholecystokinin-pancreozymin.
36 (d)
37 (c) Surgery is of no help in uncomplicated pancreatitis and should be avoided if the diagnosis is certain since the patient's general condition is likely to be poor.
38 (b) In cholecystitis, even if the gall bladder is not functioning, bile will enter the duodenum directly from the liver.
39 (d) Failure to absorb fat may be due to failure of bile to reach the duodenum (obstructive jaundice) or to deficiency of pancreatic lipase. A normal person can easily absorb 50% more fat than usual. Carbohydrate remains as such in the gut and an excess is not changed into fat until it has been absorbed.
40 (a) The common bile duct runs through the head of the pancreas and may be invaded or compressed by carcinoma there. Obstruction of the cystic duct does not cause jaundice and is rarely due to carcinoma of the pancreas.
41 (a) The diet should contain less fat than normal. To make up for the reduced intake of calories (as fat) the diet should be high in carbohydrate.
42 (b) The muscular layer is not folded. Lacteals are lymphatic channels in the villi. Goblet cells are secretory (they secrete mucus), *not* absorptive.
43 (b) The pyloric and anal sphincters control gastric and rectal emptying respectively. The mitral valve is the atrioventricular valve of the left side of the heart.
44 (b)
45 (d) Peristaltic function is provided by the muscular layer, not the mucosa.
46 (d) After fat has been emulsified by bile salts, lipase breaks it down chemically.
47 (c) Neither peptic ulcer nor peritonitis cause *colicky* pain, and in paralytic ileus the intestine is paralysed and unable to contract.
48 (c) Intestinal obstruction is the only choice which *all* the disorders may lead to as a *direct* effect of their presence.
49 (b) Kidney stones and intestinal obstruction may cause colic but not mucocele, jaundice or pancreatitis. Alcoholism may predispose to jaundice and pancreatitis but not to colic or mucocele of the gall bladder.
50 (a) In intestinal obstruction from mechanical causes (e.g.

hernia, volvulus, neoplasm), pain is colicky due to increased peristalsis attempting to overcome the obstruction, and constipation (not diarrhoea) is present.

51 (d) Treatment depends upon the cause, e.g. evacuant enema or manual removal of impacted faeces, surgery for other causes, except paralytic ileus, but *never* a purgative.

52 (b) Never give an aperient or anything by mouth to a patient suspected of having acute intestinal obstruction. Blood transfusion may not be needed.

53 (c) Enteropathy (gut disease) and sprue may *cause* steatorrhoea (fatty stools), but do not define it. Diarrhoea is the passing of unformed or frequent stools (which may or may not be associated with steatorrhoea).

54 (d) The diet should be *free* from gluten, thus wheat and rye (which contain gluten) should be avoided.

55 (b)

56 (a)

57 (a) Allergy to food is NOT a form of food poisoning. The other three choices may all cause food poisoning.

58 (b)

59 (b) While it is true that the appendix opens from the colon, since the caecum is part of the colon, the caecum is given as a choice and is the more specific answer.

60 (d) Central abdominal colicky pain is *usual*, although not invariable, *at first*.

61 (a)

62 (a)

63 (d) Peptic ulcer and hiatus hernia may bleed, but the blood is altered by digestion as it passes along the small intestine and becomes dark brown or black. Small amounts of altered blood will not be visible to the naked eye.

64 (c) There is a tendency to loose or frequent stools in hyperthyroidism.

65 (d) Abdominal pain may have medical (diabetic ketosis, herpes zoster) or surgical causes.

66 (c) Adhesions are not strong enough to cause complications until several days after operation.

67 (b) A *colo*stomy may be made for diseases of the rectum or sigmoid colon.

68 (a) Residues irritate the inflamed bowel. Protein is being lost from the ulcerated mucosa and may lead to hypoproteinaemia.

69 (a) Codeine compound contains so little codeine as to be ineffective against diarrhoea. Tincture of opium and morphine should not be used for *long-term* treatment owing to the possibility of addiction, although tincture of opium may be used for a brief period of severe diarrhoea.
70 (a) Fludrocortisone has little anti-inflammatory action.
71 (b) Inflammation of the colon is called colitis. If a diverticular pouch is inflamed it is called diverticulitis.
72 (d) Rest in bed, antibiotic, analgesic and antispasmodic cures *most* acute attacks.
73 (c)
74 (d)
75 (b) Unlike neomycin, penicillin and ampicillin are well-absorbed and do not reach the large intestinal lumen. Purgatives are likely to lead to dehydration, which is undesirable.
76 (c)
77 (c) Paralytic ileus is very common. Diarrhoea sometimes occurs.
78 (b)
79 (c)

# 9 The Liver and Biliary System

1. The normal adult liver weighs
   - (a) 1500 g
   - (b) 1100 g
   - (c) 750 g
   - (d) 250 g

2. Foreign particles in the blood flowing through the liver are taken up by
   - (a) hepatic cubical (parenchymal, main) cells (hepatocytes)
   - (b) sinusoidal Kupffer cells
   - (c) phagocytes lining the hepatic vein
   - (d) the liver does not take up foreign particles

3. One of the following is not a function of adult liver
   - (a) secretion
   - (b) excretion
   - (c) metabolism
   - (d) haemopoiesis

4. The liver does not store
   - (a) iron
   - (b) vitamins B12 and A
   - (c) bilirubin
   - (d) glycogen

5. One of the following is not synthesized by the liver
   - (a) glycogen
   - (b) prothrombin
   - (c) oestrogen
   - (d) urea

6. Vitamin K deficiency leads to a low level, in the blood, of
   - (a) bilirubin
   - (b) prothrombin
   - (c) transaminase
   - (d) platelets

7. Bilirubin is made from
   - (a) vitamin K
   - (b) prothrombin
   - (c) liver cells
   - (d) haemoglobin

8  One of the following does not cause jaundice

   (a) obstruction of the common bile duct
   (b) haemolytic anaemia
   (c) hypochromic anaemia     (d) damage to liver cells

9  In a patient with jaundice due to uncomplicated liver cell damage it is likely that the

   (a) appetite is normal and jaundice is pale
   (b) appetite is poor, and blood prothrombin level is low
   (c) serum transaminase and prothrombin levels are normal
   (d) jaundice is pronounced and greenish, the skin itches and the faeces are pale and bulky

10 In obstructive jaundice, pale and bulky faeces indicate that excess of fat is reaching the colon because

   (a) of a deficiency of pancreatic lipase
   (b) bilirubin is not being excreted into the duodenum
   (c) bile salts are not reaching the duodenum
   (d) of some reason other than those mentioned above

11 A common cause of liver damage is

   (a) virus hepatitis     (b) leptospirosis
   (c) toluene poisoning
   (d) hair shampoos containing selenium

12 Virus hepatitis is not due to

   (a) infective hepatitis (virus A) or serum hepatitis (virus B)
   (b) glandular fever     (c) yellow fever     (d) typhoid fever

13 The treatment of infective hepatitis is rest and a

   (a) high protein, high calorie diet and to forbid alcohol
   (b) high carbohydrate diet, including alcohol
   (c) high calorie diet and sedation with phenobarbitone
   (d) low calorie, low-fat diet and give gamma-globulin

# Liver and Biliary System

14 Cirrhosis of the liver is

   (a) hardening of the liver by fibrosis
   (b) fatty deposition in the liver
   (c) a form of carcinoma
   (d) the change occurring during acute hepatitis

15 One of the following does not cause hepatic cirrhosis

   (a) alcoholism        (b) excessive iron or copper deposition
   (c) biliary disease   (d) portal hypertension

16 In hepatic failure with disturbed brain function (encephalopathy) the diet should be low in

   (a) salt    (b) fat    (c) protein    (d) carbohydrate

17 Obstructive jaundice is not due to

   (a) a gall stone in the common bile duct
   (b) carcinoma of the head of the pancreas
   (c) obstruction of small bile ducts in the liver
   (d) cholecystitis

18 The history, degree of jaundice, bruising, itching, vomitus and the colour, quantity and odour of the faeces are all important observations in

   (a) obstructive jaundice      (b) haemolytic jaundice
   (c) hepatocellular damage     (d) all forms of jaundice

19 If vomitus contains bile it indicates that any jaundice is

   (a) obstructive    (b) not obstructive
   (c) haemolytic     (d) viral in origin

20 The absence of bile in vomitus indicates

   (a) biliary obstruction      (b) absence of biliary obstruction
   (c) pyloric stenosis
   (d) that bile is not regurgitating into the stomach

21 One of the following is not a function of the gall bladder

   (a) secretion of bile        (b) storage of bile
   (c) concentration of bile    (d) secretion of mucus

22 The process of emulsification of fat (by bile) is

   (a) a chemical (enzymatic) breakdown of fat to fatty acids
   (b) a physical breakdown to small globules of fat
   (c) both     (d) neither

23 At 6 p.m. on the day before cholecystography, the patient is given a fatty meal in order to

   (a) empty the gall bladder     (b) test gall bladder function
   (c) test liver function        (d) all of these

24 In acute cholecystitis pain is mainly in the

   (a) left hypochondrium     (b) right hypochondrium
   (c) left hypochondrium, radiating to the left shoulder
   (d) left iliac fossa

25 Which of the following does not occur in acute cholecystitis?

   (a) pyrexia     (b) pain     (c) jaundice     (d) vomiting

26 The early treatment of acute cholecystitis may be with

   (a) intragastric drip, antibiotic and antispasmodic
   (b) morphine for pain, antibiotic and fat-free diet
   (c) antibiotic, pethidine, antispasmodic, and fat-free diet or intravenous drip
   (d) antibiotic, intravenous drip and fat-free diet

27 Gallstones consist largely of

   (a) calcium        (b) bile salts
   (c) cholesterol    (d) phosphates

28 If gall stones are present, they

   (a) always produce symptoms
   (b) always produce complications
   (c) always cause both symptoms and complications
   (d) may never cause symptoms or complications

29 Which of the following is not a complication of gall stones?

   (a) obstruction of the cystic duct     (b) mucocele
   (c) haematemesis
   (d) obstruction of the common bile duct

# Liver and Biliary System

30 Obstructive jaundice due to gall stones is treated by
  (a) operation      (b) diet
  (c) drugs          (d) diet, drugs and rest

31 Opening the common bile duct to remove a stone is called
  (a) cholecystectomy    (b) cholecystostomy
  (c) choledochotomy     (d) cholecystography

32 A T-drainage tube is used to drain the
  (a) common bile duct   (b) bladder
  (c) gall bladder       (d) gall bladder bed

# Answers

1 (a)
2 (b) Hepatic sinusoids are lined with phagocytic reticulo-endothelial (Kupffer) cells which take up foreign particles e.g. bacteria, from the blood received through the portal vein. Hepatocytes are not phagocytic. The hepatic vein is not lined with phagocytes.
3 (d)
4 (c) The liver metabolises and excretes bilirubin.
5 (c) Oestrogen is made by the ovaries and adrenal cortex.
6 (b) The liver manufactures prothrombin from vitamin K.
7 (d) The haemoglobin of old red blood cells is broken down and the haem is changed to bilirubin which is excreted into the bile by the liver.
8 (c) In hypochromic anaemia the rate of red cells breakdown is not increased, unlike haemolytic anaemia in which haemolysis leads to increased bilirubin production. Damaged liver cells cannot excrete bilirubin, and obstruction of the common bile duct prevents bile (and hence bilirubin) from leaving the liver, thus bilirubin levels build up in the blood.

9  (b) The symptoms described in (a) and (c) describe haemolytic jaundice, and those in (d) are found in obstructive jaundice. Liver damage may be complicated by intrahepatic obstruction, but the question stated that the liver damage was uncomplicated.
10 (c) Deficiency of bile salts in the duodenum, owing to obstruction of the common bile duct, leads to failure of emulsification of fat. Fat has to be emulsified before pancreatic lipase can hydrolyse it for absorption. Fat therefore remains in the gut and produces pale and bulky faeces. Bilirubin is merely a waste product which is excreted in the bile and is unrelated to fat absorption.
11 (a) The other choices may cause liver damage, but *not* commonly—the question asked for a *common* cause.
12 (d) Hepatitis viruses A and B, glandular fever and yellow fever are all viruses which may cause hepatitis.
13 (a) Alcohol is toxic to the liver and should be forbidden. Gamma-globulin is useless as *therapy* but may be given *before* symptoms appear in an attempt to attenuate the disease.
14 (a) Hepatic cirrhosis does not occur *during* acute hepatitis, but may follow it as a complication.
15 (d) Portal hypertension is a result, not a cause of hepatic cirrhosis.
16 (c) Protein breakdown products worsen the encephalopathy. The diet should be *high* in carbohydrate so as to reduce protein breakdown.
Salt is restricted if there is ascites, but ascites was not part of the question.
17 (d)
18 (d)
19 (b) Bile stained vomit indicates that bile is reaching the duodenum, therefore there cannot be obstruction to the common bile duct.
20 (d) The absence of bile in vomitus merely means that bile is not regurgitating from the duodenum into the stomach. Bile may therefore be absent from the vomit, even when it is present in the duodenum. Bile does not regurgitate in the normal person.
21 (a) Bile is *secreted* only by the liver.
22 (b) Fat is broken into tiny globules (emulsified) so as to increase its surface area. This is *followed* by enzymatic breakdown by lipase, producing fatty acids.

# Liver and Biliary System

23 (a) The gall bladder has to be emptied so as to allow it to fill with radio-opaque 'dye'.
24 (b) Pain occurs in the *right* hypochondrium (and may radiate to the *right* shoulder).
25 (c) Jaundice is not a sign of cholecystitis. If jaundice is present it is due to some complication such as cholangitis or a gall stone in the common bile duct.
26 (c) Morphine and pethidine contract the biliary sphincter (of Oddi) and should not be used unless an antispasmodic is also given. The stomach should be kept empty by gastric aspiration to subdue hormonal (cholecystokinin) stimulation of the gall bladder. An intravenous drip is used for the first 3 to 5 days, *followed by* a fat-free diet once symptoms have subsided.
27 (c) Gall stones often also contain bile *pigment*, and *may* contain *small amounts* of calcium.
28 (d) Gall stones may cause symptoms, but may be 'silent', i.e. present but symptomless.
29 (c) Obstruction of the cystic duct is a cause of mucocele and of cholecystitis.
30 (a) Cholecystectomy and opening the common bile duct to remove stone(s) from it.
31 (c)
32 (a)

# 10 The Urinary System

1. The nephron consists of a
   - (a) whole kidney
   - (b) glomerulus and its tubule
   - (c) glomerulus only
   - (d) glomerulus, tubule and renal pelvis

2. Blood enters the glomerulus through
   - (a) the afferent arteriole
   - (b) the efferent arteriole
   - (c) the juxtaglomerular apparatus
   - (d) the proximal tubule

3. The glomerular filtrate is produced by
   - (a) osmotic pressure
   - (b) blood pressure
   - (c) diffusion
   - (d) secretion

4. The glomerular filtrate consists of
   - (a) plasma
   - (b) serum
   - (c) plasma without its large (protein) molecules
   - (d) serum without its small molecules

5. The amount of glomerular filtrate re-absorbed by the tubules is approximately
   - (a) 99%
   - (b) 50%
   - (c) 18%
   - (d) 1.5%

6. The action of antidiuretic hormone is to
   - (a) increase the concentration of salt outside the tubule
   - (b) decrease the concentration of salt inside the tubule
   - (c) decrease tubular re-absorption of water
   - (d) increase tubular re-absorption of water

7. Hydrocortisone and aldosterone are secreted by the
   - (a) renal cortex
   - (b) renal medulla
   - (c) adrenal medulla
   - (d) adrenal cortex

# Urinary System

8  Hydrocortisone and aldosterone increase
   (a) urinary output    (b) tubular re-absorption of sodium
   (c) tubular re-absorption of potassium
   (d) all of these

9  Certain cells, near the glomeruli of the kidney (juxtaglomerular cells), secrete a substance which leads to an increase in blood pressure. This substance is
   (a) rennin           (b) renin
   (c) angiotensinogen  (d) angiotensin

10 Functions of the kidneys include
   (a) control of acid-base balance
   (b) stimulation of red cell production
   (c) metabolism of vitamin D    (d) all of these

11 Failure of the kidneys to produce any urine is called
   (a) retention of urine   (b) anuria
   (c) oliguria             (d) polyuria

12 One of the following is not a cause of haematuria
   (a) renal colic     (b) bladder tumour
   (c) renal stones    (d) cystitis

13 Proteinuria is least likely to occur in
   (a) mild exertion   (b) pyelonephritis
   (c) cystitis        (d) congestive cardiac failure

14 Ketonuria does not result from
   (a) starvation   (b) diabetes mellitus
   (c) nephritis    (d) vomiting

15 The reaction (pH) of normal urine is
   (a) slightly alkaline   (b) slightly acid
   (c) neutral             (d) very alkaline

16 The normal volume of urine in 24 hours averages

   (a) 500 to 1000 ml      (b) 1000 to 1600 ml
   (c) 1600 to 2500 ml     (d) over 2.5 l

17 Bacterial infection of the kidney, e.g. complicating cystitis, is called

   (a) glomerulonephritis     (b) pyelonephritis
   (c) nephrotic syndrome     (d) enuresis

18 The treatment of acute glomerulonephritis is

   (a) antibiotic, diuretic and azathioprine
   (b) rest in bed, low protein diet, diuretic, azathioprine
   (c) rest in bed, salt, fluid and protein restriction, and penicillin for the kidney
   (d) rest in bed, salt, fluid and protein restriction, and penicillin for a sore throat

19 A patient with pain in the loins, rigors, pyrexia, vomiting, and pus and organisms in the urine is likely to be suffering from

   (a) acute nephritis      (b) nephrotic syndrome
   (c) renal infection      (d) hydronephrosis

20 An essential sign of the nephrotic syndrome is

   (a) haematuria                  (b) pus in the urine
   (c) albuminuria and oedema      (d) all of the above

21 A common cause of the nephrotic syndrome is

   (a) amyloidosis          (b) thrombosis of the renal vein
   (c) mercury poisoning    (d) quartan malaria

22 The dietary treatment of the early stage of the nephrotic syndrome is likely to be

   (a) high protein     (b) low protein
   (c) high salt        (d) low carbohydrate

# Urinary System

23 Severe shock, incompatible blood transfusion, acute nephritis, acute pancreatitis and myocardial infarction may all cause

(a) acute pyelonephritis  (b) chronic glomerulonephritis
(c) acute renal failure  (d) hydronephrosis

24 Prednisolone produces a rapid relief from oedema in

(a) acute glomerulonephritis  (b) chronic nephritis
(c) cardio-renal failure  (d) nephrotic syndrome

25 The treatment of acute renal failure is

(a) intravenous fluid and electrolytes
(b) blood transfusion
(c) plasma  (d) dependent on the cause

26 Osteodystrophy, pericarditis, arrhythmias, convulsions and anaemia are all complications of

(a) acute renal failure  (b) hypernephroma
(c) chronic renal failure  (d) acute pyelonephritis

27 Renal stones never consist of

(a) calcium oxalate  (b) calcium phosphate
(c) uric acid  (d) cholesterol

28 Ureteric colic is due to

(a) the pain of a stone abrading the mucosa of the ureter
(b) reflex pain caused by frequency of micturition
(c) smooth muscle spasm  (d) dilatation of the ureter

29 The treatment of ureteric colic is

(a) morphine, atropine and liberal fluids
(b) pethidine and alkali
(c) propantheline, alkali and liberal fluids
(d) immediate surgical removal if the stone is small

30 Most renal stones are due to

(a) renal infection
(b) excessive intake of calcium (milk) and alkali
(c) gout  (d) hyperparathyroidism

31 The urge to pass urine every few minutes, but only a few drops are passed, with difficulty, as in ureteric colic, is called

(a) urgency (b) strangury
(c) incontinence (d) tenesmus

32 Polyuria, nocturia, dehydration, thirst and uraemia are likely to be due to

(a) chronic renal failure (b) acute renal failure
(c) unilateral hydronephrosis (d) bladder carcinoma

33 In uraemia due to chronic renal failure, a suitable daily diet may contain

(a) fat 65 g, carbohydrate 300 g, protein 20 to 40 g
(b) fat 50 g, carbohydrate 80 g, protein 30 g
(c) fat 100 g, carbohydrate 80 g, no protein
(d) fat 50 g, carbohydrate 250 g, protein 20 g, high potassium

34 After a renal transplant the patient is barrier-nursed because

(a) he may spread infection to visitors
(b) the transplant may be infected
(c) the blood transfusions he has received may have given him hepatitis
(d) he may become infected because of the drug therapy he is receiving

35 Dilatation of the renal calyces and pelvis is called

(a) hydrocephalus (b) hydronephrosis
(c) mucocele (d) varicocele

36 Dilatation of the renal pelvis may be due to

(a) calculi or tumours
(b) stricture of the ureter or urethra
(c) both (a) and (b) (d) neither (a) nor (b)

37 Polycystic disease of the kidneys is due to

(a) a genetic abnormality (b) hypertension
(c) senility (d) chronic cystitis

# Urinary System

38 The insertion of a tube into the kidney is called

(a) nephrolithotomy  (b) pyelolithotomy
(c) nephrostomy  (d) nephrectomy

39 The operation to correct hydronephrosis is called

(a) pyloroplasty  (b) pyeloplasty
(c) ureterostomy  (d) cystostomy

40 A tissue taken from and grafted into the same person is an

(a) autograft  (b) homograft
(c) allograft  (d) xenograft

41 A perinephric abscess is an abscess

(a) in the renal medulla  (b) in the renal cortex
(c) outside the kidney but beneath its fatty capsule
(d) outside the perirenal fatty capsule

42 Before an operation on the kidney it is necessary to

(a) transfuse the patient with blood
(b) wash out the bladder
(c) give iron  (d) empty the bowel and bladder

43 After a renal operation the tube in the perinephric space is usually removed on the

(a) first day  (b) third day
(c) seventh day  (d) tenth day

44 In what position does the prostate lie in relation to the urinary bladder?

(a) in front  (b) below  (c) behind  (d) above

45 How many orifices are there in the bladder

(a) one  (b) two  (c) three  (d) four

46 Before cystoscopy in the male

   (a) the suprapubic area is shaved
   (b) the bladder should be emptied
   (c) fluid intake is limited
   (d) the suprapubic area need not be shaved

47 Incontinence of urine is due to

   (a) overactivity of the detrusor muscle
   (b) weakness of the urinary sphincters
   (c) both (a) and (b)    (d) neither (a) nor (b)

48 Acute retention of urine may be caused by

   (a) operations on the rectum and anus
   (b) prostatic enlargement, phimosis, urethal stricture
   (c) lesions of the nervous system such as tabes or multiple sclerosis
   (d) all of the above

49 Catheterisation of the urinary bladder

   (a) is so simple and safe that it does not cause complications
   (b) may cause cystitis
   (c) may cause urethritis, cystitis, meatal stricture or ulceration
   (d) always leads to cystitis

50 Before passing a catheter into the urinary bladder

   (a) chlorhexidine should be put into the urethra
   (b) lignocaine 1% with chlorhexidine should be put into the urethra
   (c) nothing should be put into the urethra so as not to contaminate it
   (d) chlorhexidine should be put into the catheter

51 The treatment of both haematuria with clot formation and chronic cystitis may be

   (a) bladder lavage or irrigation    (b) antibiotic
   (c) catheterisation    (d) diathermy

52 Endoscopic resection, cystodiothermy, megavoltage radiotherapy, and partial or total cystectomy are all types of treatment for
   (a) carcinoma of the kidney  (b) carcinoma of the bladder
   (c) benign papilloma of the bladder
   (d) carcinoma of the prostate

# Answers

1 (b)
2 (a) Afferent means to carry toward (ad = toward, ferre = carry).
   Efferent means to carry away or outward (ex = out).
3 (b) The glomerular filtrate is produced by mechanical (hydrostatic) blood pressure.
4 (c) Water and small molecules (glucose, electrolytes, amino acids, urea, etc.) are filtered from the plasma into the renal tubules. Large molecules, such as protein, remain in the blood capillaries.
5 (a) The daily glomerular filtrate is normally 180 l. 178.5 l is re-absorbed, 1.5 l is excreted as urine.
6 (d)
7 (d)
8 (b) Hydrocortisone and aldosterone increase the tubular re-absorption of sodium, but decrease the re-absorption of potassium, i.e. sodium leaves the tubule partly in exchange for potassium. When more sodium is re-absorbed water re-absorption automatically follows, therefore urinary output tends to decrease.
9 (b) Renin converts angiotensinogen (present in the plasma) into angiotensin, which increases blood pressure. Rennin is the enzyme, secreted by the stomach, which clots milk.

10 (d)
11 (b) In urinary retention, urine is produced by the kidneys and collects in the bladder but cannot be voided, e.g. because of obstruction by an enlarged prostate. Oliguria and pulyuria are diminished and increased urine production respectively.
12 (a) Renal colic is a symptom, not a disease.
13 (a)
14 (c) Ketosis *may* result from starvation, diabetes mellitus or vomiting.
15 (b) The normal pH of urine is about 6.0 (slightly acid).
16 (b)
17 (b)
18 (d) Azathioprine is ineffective. The kidney is not infected therefore choice (c) is incorrect. Acute nephritis is commonly preceded by a streptococcal sore throat, if this is still present penicillin is advisable.
19 (c) These are the classical symptoms and signs of renal infection.
20 (c) Haematuria is often absent and pus is not a feature.
21 (d) The other three choices are *rare* causes; the question asks for a common cause.
22 (a) The oedema is due to hypoproteinaemia, therefore a high protein diet is given unless there is renal failure (which is rare in the *early* stages).
Salt intake should be restricted.
23 (c)
24 (d) Prednisolone would make the oedema *worse* in cardio-renal failure and often also in acute nephritis, owing to further salt and water retention.
25 (d) Intravenous fluid and electrolytes are given for acute renal failure (ARF) due to Addison's disease or heat stroke, but the correct treatment for ARF due to haemorrhage is blood transfusion.
In anuria electrolytes are not being lost and are not required. The treatment therefore, differs for each of the many causes of acute renal failure.
26 (c) Osteodystrophy takes months or years to develop.
It is not due to acute or unilateral conditions.
27 (d) It is *gall stones* which contain cholesterol.
28 (c) The ureteric smooth muscle contracts in spasm around the stone or blood clot in the lumen. The mucosa is not sensitive to pain.

# Urinary System

29 (a) Alkali decreases the solubility of calcium and is therefore undesirable where the calculi consist of calcium. A *small* stone is treated expectantly since many will be passed spontaneously. Surgery may be needed, but not immediately.

30 (a) The other 3 choices may also lead to calculi but *most* stones are due to renal infection.

31 (b) Strangos (Greek) = a drop, ouron = urine. Tenesmos = straining.

32 (a)

33 (a) This supplies approximately 2000 kcal (8.4 MJ), sufficient to prevent excessive breakdown of tissue protein. 80 g of carbohydrate is inadequate. Potassium is retained in renal failure, leading to hyperkalaemia and possible cardiac dysrhythmia. The diet should, therefore, be *low* in potassium.

34 (d) The patient receives immunosuppressive drugs in order to prevent him from producing an immune response, e.g. antibodies, against the foreign kidney. These drugs also suppress his immunity to infection.

35 (b)

36 (c)

37 (a) It is an autosomal dominant trait.

38 (c)

39 (b)

40 (a) A homograft (allograft) is tissue taken from another individual of the same species; a xenograft is from a different species.

41 (c)

42 (d) Iron or blood transfusion may or may not be necessary, but the bowel and bladder should always be emptied.

43 (b) In the absence of complications, the tube is removed on the third day.

44 (b)

45 (c) Two ureters and the urethra.

46 (d) The patient should drink freely so that, at cystoscopy, urine can be observed coming from each ureteric orifice, and the bladder should be fairly full.

47 (c)

48 (d)

49 (c) Catheterisation has risks, but these are reduced by careful technique.

50 (b) The urethra should first be anaesthetised.

51 (a) An antibiotic may be given for chronic cystitis but not for *both*.
Diathermy may be used to destroy a bleeding papilloma but not for chronic cystitis.
52 (b)

# 11 The Reproductive System

1 The germinal epithelial cells of the testis produce spermatozoa when stimulated by

   (a) follicle-stimulating hormone    (b) corticotrophin
   (c) oxytocin    (d) adrenaline

2 The interstitial cells of the testis secrete

   (a) oestrogen    (b) gonadotrophin
   (c) testosterone    (d) all of these

3 Epididymo-orchitis is not due to

   (a) trauma    (b) mumps
   (c) spread of infection from a urethritis
   (d) spread of infection from a salpingitis

4 The inner lining of the uterine wall consists of

   (a) endometrium    (b) endothelium
   (c) myometrium    (d) peritoneum

5 The free end of the fallopian tube

   (a) is closed    (b) opens into the peritoneal cavity
   (c) opens into the uterus
   (d) opens into the ovary

6 The ovary produces

   (a) ova    (b) oestrogen
   (c) progesterone    (d) ova, oestrogen and progesterone

7 A substantial amount of oestrogen is produced by the ovarian

   (a) follicle    (b) corpus luteum
   (c) corpus albicans    (d) all of these

8 Ovarian function is controlled by the following hormone(s)

  (a) follicle-stimulating  (b) luteinising
  (c) follicle-stimulating and luteinising
  (d) follicle-stimulating, luteinising and oxytocin

9 The dormant ova in the ovary are called

  (a) Graafian follicles  (b) primordial follicles
  (c) spores  (d) corpus callosum

10 Fertilisation occurs in the

  (a) vagina  (b) uterus  (c) fallopian tube  (d) ovary

11 The treatment of preference for benign prostatic hypertrophy in a fit patient is

  (a) radiotherapy  (b) chemotherapy
  (c) indwelling catheter  (d) prostatectomy

12 After prostatectomy for benign prostatic hypertrophy, one of the following does not apply:

  (a) oestrogen is given  (b) high fluid intake is needed
  (c) watch for bleeding  (d) urethral stricture may occur

13 If clot retention follows prostatectomy, the bladder may be irrigated with a solution of

  (a) sodium bicarbonate  (b) sodium citrate
  (c) warfarin (anticoagulant)  (d) antibiotic

14 The treatment of phimosis is

  (a) dorsal slit  (b) dilatation with bougies
  (c) circumcision  (d) sterilisation

15 Fibroadenosis of the breast is due to

  (a) benign neoplasm (tumour)  (b) malignant neoplasm
  (c) trauma  (d) hormonal imbalance

# Reproductive System

16 A discharge from the nipple, due to a simple cyst of the breast is

   (a) bloodstained     (b) clear and thin
   (c) green or brown     (d) milky

17 A carcinomatous nodule of the breast

   (a) is smooth and painful     (b) never ulcerates
   (c) does not spread via the lymphatics
   (d) is painless and irregular

18 For the first 24 hours after mastectomy a careful watch must be kept

   (a) for haemorrhage     (b) for recurrence of carcinoma
   (c) for oozing of serum
   (d) to make sure that the patient performs full arm exercises

19 During and for life bilateral adrenalectomy for carcinoma of the breast the patient receives

   (a) morphine     (b) cortisone
   (c) thyroxine     (d) corticotrophin (ACTH)

## Answers

1 (a) Follicle-stimulating hormone, secreted by the pituitary, stimulates the germinal epithelial cells of the testis in the male, and the ovary in the female.
2 (c)
3 (d) Salpingitis is inflammation of the fallopian tubes—which are absent from the male.
4 (a) Endothelium is the inner lining (intima) of blood vessels. Myometrium is the middle (muscular) layer of the uterus, the outer layer of the fundus and body of the uterus being peritoneum.

5 (b)
6 (d) While choices (a), (b) and (c) are true, choice (d) is the more informative and is therefore the correct one.
7 (a) The corpus luteum produces progesterone. The corpus albicans (the degenerate corpus luteum) does not produce any hormone.
8 (c) Oxytocin produces uterine contractions.
9 (b) The ova in the Graafian follicles are no longer *dormant*.
10 (c)
11 (d) An indwelling catheter is used only if the patient's condition is poor.
12 (a) Oestrogen is used in *carcinoma* of the prostate, not in benign hypertrophy.
13 (b) A solution of 3.8% sodium citrate prevents clotting.
14 (c)
15 (d) Fibroadenosis is not a true neoplasm (tumour).
16 (b) A discharge is likely to be bloodstained in carcinoma, green or brown in fibroadenosis, or milky after lactation.
17 (d) Carcinoma of the breast is irregular, painless, ulcerates, and spreads via the lymphatics.
18 (a) Recurrence of carcinoma will not be seen until weeks or months later.
   Oozing of serum is expected in the first 24 hours. Arm movements are commenced (gradually) on the *second* day.
19 (b) Cortisone is changed in the body to cortisol, one of the hormones which is essential for life, secreted by the adrenal cortex. Giving corticotrophin is useless after adrenalectomy, since there are no adrenals for it to stimulate!

# 12 The Endocrine System

1. The endocrine glands are controlled by the
   - (a) posterior lobe of the pituitary
   - (b) hypothalamus
   - (c) cerebellum
   - (d) pituitary fossa

2. The pituitary gland is attached by a stalk to the
   - (a) thyroid
   - (b) thalamus
   - (c) hypothalamus
   - (d) pineal

3. The posterior lobe of the pituitary stores or secretes
   - (a) vasopressin
   - (b) progesterone
   - (c) growth hormone
   - (d) follicle-stimulating hormone

4. The anterior lobe of the pituitary does not secrete one of the following
   - (a) thyrotrophin
   - (b) somatotrophin
   - (c) prolactin
   - (d) oxytocin

5. The adrenal glands are stimulated by
   - (a) corticotrophin
   - (b) prolactin
   - (c) luteinising hormone
   - (d) calcitonin

6. The alpha ($\alpha$)-cells of the pancreatic islets secrete
   - (a) adrenaline
   - (b) glucagon
   - (c) insulin
   - (d) calcitonin

7. The secretion of antidiuretic hormone (ADH) is directly controlled by the
   - (a) kidney
   - (b) osmoreceptors
   - (c) adrenal cortex
   - (d) insulin

8. Prolactin causes the secretion of
   - (a) calcitonin
   - (b) properdin
   - (c) urine
   - (d) milk

9 Progesterone is secreted by the

   (a) corpus luteum
   (b) corpus albicans
   (c) primordial follicles
   (d) anterior pituitary

10 In diabetes insipidus, deficiency of antidiuretic hormone leads to

   (a) anuria
   (b) oliguria
   (c) polyuria
   (d) a normal urinary volume

11 Acromegaly is due to an excess of

   (a) thyroxine
   (b) growth hormone in childhood
   (c) growth hormone in adults
   (d) parathyroid hormone

12 Panhypopituitarism (Simmond's disease) is treated with

   (a) insulin
   (b) insulin and thyroxine
   (c) thyroxine alone
   (d) cortisone, thyroxine and sex hormone

13 Behind the thyroid gland there are

   (a) adrenals and nerves
   (b) adrenals and trachea
   (c) two parathyroid glands
   (d) four parathyroid glands

14 The thyroid gland stores

   (a) thyrotrophin
   (b) thyroglobulin
   (c) cortisol
   (d) none of these

15 The thyroid secretes the hormones

   (a) thyroglobulin
   (b) thyroxine and thyroglobulin
   (c) thyroxine and calcitonin
   (d) calcitonin and cortisol

16 A goitre is always due to

   (a) thyrotoxicosis
   (b) an enlarged lymph node in the neck
   (c) an enlarged salivary gland
   (d) an enlarged thyroid gland

# Endocrine System

17 Hyperthyroidism may be due to

   (a) toxic adenoma of the thyroid
   (b) Graves' disease (exophthalmic goitre)
   (c) neither    (d) both

18 Loss of weight, a moist cold skin, fine tremor, and a pulse rate which is increased during the day but normal during sleep, is likely to be caused by

   (a) hyperthyroidism    (b) anxiety state
   (c) neither of these    (d) both of these

19 One of the following is not a form of treatment for hyperthyroidism

   (a) digoxin    (b) antithyroid drugs
   (c) radioactive iodine    (d) surgery

20 A patient receiving carbimazole (Neomercazole) is told that she should report any sore throat immediately to her doctor because she may have

   (a) agranulocytosis    (b) thyrotoxicosis
   (c) dermatitis    (d) cardiac failure

21 In hyperthyroidism the diet should commonly be

   (a) high in coffee content    (b) low in calories
   (c) low in protein    (d) high in calories and protein

22 The initial daily treatment of a patient with severe hypothyroidism is

   (a) carbimazole 30 mg    (b) thyroxine 3 mg or more
   (c) thyroxine 0.3 mg    (d) thyroxine 0.05 mg or less

23 Hypothyroidism in childhood is called

   (a) gargoylism    (b) cretinism
   (c) thyroiditis    (d) hypothermia

24 Parathyroid hormone controls the metabolism of

   (a) sodium and potassium    (b) calcium and phosphate
   (c) the thyroid    (d) the adrenals

25 Tetany is a form of

(a) muscular spasm  (b) tetanus infection
(c) hyperthyroidism  (d) hyperparathyroidism

26 The adrenal glands consist of

(a) an inner cortex and outer medulla
(b) a cortex of sympathetic cells
(c) an inner medulla and outer cortex
(d) none of these

27 The adrenal cortex secretes

(a) adrenaline  (b) noradrenaline
(c) antidiuretic hormone  (d) cortisol and aldosterone

28 Dehydration and low blood pressure due to loss of sodium, chloride and water in the urine, may be due to

(a) Addison's disease (hypoadrenocorticism)
(b) hyperthyroidism
(c) Cushing's syndrome (hyperadrenocortism)
(d) hypothyroidism

29 Cushing's syndrome is not due to

(a) pituitary tumour  (b) adrenal cortical tumour
(c) adrenal medullary tumour  (d) corticosteroid therapy

30 Adrenal corticosteroid therapy, e.g. prednisolone, may cause

(a) diabetes mellitus  (b) hypertension
(c) osteoporosis  (d) all of these

31 Adrenal corticosteroid therapy may lead to

(a) cardiac failure  (b) adrenal atrophy
(c) infection  (d) all of these

32 The blood glucose ('sugar') is controlled by

(a) insulin  (b) glucagon
(c) both of these  (d) neither of these

# Endocrine System

33 Symptoms in untreated diabetes mellitus do not include

   (a) polyuria         (b) glycosuria
   (c) hypoglycaemia    (d) ketosis

34 Diabetics are not more liable than average to suffer from

   (a) infections              (b) ischaemic heart disease
   (c) congenital heart disease (d) cataract and neuropathy

35 Diabetics have glycosuria because they have

   (a) a high blood glucose level
   (b) a low renal threshold for glucose
   (c) a high renal threshold for glucose
   (d) too much insulin

36 The diet in patients with diabetes mellitus should be

   (a) low in calories (energy)    (b) high in protein and fat
   (c) low in energy (calories) and fat
   (d) some other diet

37 In the 'adult' (obesity, 'maturity-onset') type of diabetes mellitus adequate treatment is often

   (a) low-calorie diet alone
   (b) antidiabetic tablets without controlling diet
   (c) insulin alone
   (d) high doses of insulin with a high calorie diet

38 In diabetes, non-starchy vegetables are

   (a) unrestricted        (b) restricted to small quantities
   (c) not permitted       (d) restricted to average quantities

39 A diabetic who is going to perform severe exercise, additional to that normally taken, should on that day, take

   (a) more insulin     (b) less insulin
   (c) the same amount of insulin as usual
   (d) additional antidiabetic tablets

40 Oral hypoglycaemic drugs

   (a) are completely safe     (b) may produce hypoglycaemia
   (c) may precipitate a skin rash but do not produce hypoglycaemia
   (d) may be complicated only by agranulocytosis or a skin rash

41 Pregnant women with poorly controlled diabetes are more likely than non-diabetics, to have

   (a) stillbirths     (b) large babies
   (c) neither of these
   (d) stillbirths, abortions, and large babies

42 In diabetic coma the patient requires, in the first 12 hours,

   (a) lente insulin and 4 l of fluid
   (b) soluble insulin and 2 l of fluid
   (c) soluble insulin and 6 l of fluid
   (d) the type of insulin is not important

43 In hypoglycaemic coma the following amount of glucose should be given immediately intravenously

   (a) 5 g     (b) 1 g     (c) 25 g     (d) 20 mg

# Answers

1 (b) The *posterior* lobe of the pituitary (although it secretes 2 hormones) does not control any endocrine glands, unlike the anterior lobe.
2 (c)
3 (a) Vasopressin is the antidiuretic hormone.
4 (d) Oxytocin is secreted by the *posterior* lobe of the pituitary.

# Endocrine System

5. (a) Corticotrophin (adrenocorticotrophin, ACTH) stimulates cortisol secretion by the adrenal cortex.
6. (b) The beta ($\beta$)-cells secrete insulin.
7. (b) Osmoreceptors in the hypothalamus detect concentration or dilution of the plasma and adjust ADH secretion accordingly.
8. (d) Prolactin (lactogenic hormone) induces milk secretion after childbirth.
   Before delivery it maintains the corpus luteum.
9. (a)
10. (c) Antidiuretic hormone causes the re-absorption of water from the renal tubules. Deficiency leads to failure of re-absorption of water which is therefore excreted, leading to an excessive urinary output (polyuria), dehydration and thirst.
11. (c) Excess of growth hormone in childhood leads to giantism.
12. (d) In panhypopituitarism there is deficiency of all the anterior pituitary hormones—corticotrophin, thyrotrophin, gonadotrophins and growth hormone. Cortisone and thyroxine are essential for life, and androgen or oestrogen improve health.
13. (d)
14. (b) Thyroglobulin is the storage form of the thyroid hormones. Thyrotrophin is the thyroid stimulating hormone secreted by the pituitary.
15. (c) The thyroid secretes the hormones thyroxine and calcitonin (and also tri-iodothyronine). Thyroglobulin itself is not a *hormone* but is the *precursor* of hormones.
16. (d) A goitre is an enlarged thyroid gland. It *may* be due to thyrotoxicosis, but there are other causes of thyroid enlargement, e.g. simple goitre due to iodine deficiency.
17. (d)
18. (b) In hyperthyroidism the skin is likely to be warm, and the pulse rate remains high during sleep, hence the importance of counting the sleeping pulse rate.
19. (a) Digoxin is used for certain complications of hyperthyroidism, e.g. cardiac failure, but not for hyperthyroidism itself.
20. (a) Carbimazole may cause agranulocytosis (a lack of polymorphs), thus allowing infection—commonly a throat infection, although a more serious infection is likely to follow.

21 (d) Most patients with hyperthyroidism will have lost weight and muscle protein.
Coffee has many of the actions of thyroxine and should not be taken in excess.
22 (d) Carbimazole (Neomercazole) is used in *hyper*thyroidism. The *initial* dose of thyroxine is 0.025 or 0.05 mg (25 or 50 µg) daily for two weeks, increasing gradually. Larger doses may cause lethal cardiac failure.
23 (b)
24 (b)
25 (a) Tetany is muscular spasm due to a low concentration of ionised calcium in the plasma.
26 (c) The inner part is the medulla, consisting of sympathetic cells. The outer part is the cortex.
27 (d) The *medulla* secretes adrenaline and noradrenaline.
28 (a) In Addison's disease, deficiency of aldosterone and cortisol leads to loss of salt and water in the urine, hence dehydration.
29 (c) A tumour of the adrenal medulla produces catecholamines, e.g. adrenaline, not corticosteroids.
30 (d) The choice of (a), (b) or (c) indicates that the student did not know the other two complications, and a mark is lost.
31 (d)
32 (c) Insulin lowers, and glucagon raises, the blood glucose level.
33 (c) *Un*treated diabetics have hyperglycaemia not hypoglycaemia.
34 (c) Diabetics are prone to infection, atheroma, cataract and neuropathy.
35 (a) The renal threshold for glucose is usually the same in diabetes mellitus as in the general population.
36 (d) The energy (calorie) content depends on the patient's weight. The aim is to bring the body weight to normal. In an obese diabetic, calories should be restricted, but in a juvenile diabetic, weight has usually been lost and the calorie intake should be relatively high.
37 (a) A low-energy diet, if adhered to, is often sufficient to control the diabetes. If antidiabetic tablets or insulin are used, dietary control is still necessary.
38 (a) *Non*-starchy vegetables do not supply calories and may help to satisfy appetite.
39 (b) *Less* insulin or more calories will be needed, but the

# Endocrine System

latter was not offered as part of the question. The patient would be likely to become hypoglycaemic if his usual diet and insulin were taken.

40 (b) They may lead to hypoglycaemia, and even to hypoglycaemic coma.

41 (d)

42 (c) In diabetic coma the patient is dehydrated, usually having lost about 6 l of fluid. Only soluble insulin should be used since it is the most rapidly acting and provides the easiest control of the diabetes.

43 (c) 15 to 25 g is a reasonable quantity to give as a first dose. Note that in (d) the weight is given in mg—a useless amount.

# 13 The Nervous System

1 Cerebrospinal fluid is produced by
   (a) arachnoid granulations   (b) choroid plexuses
   (c) venous sinuses   (d) the brachial plexus

2 The cerebrospinal fluid lies between the
   (a) brain and pia mater
   (b) pia mater and arachnoid mater
   (c) arachnoid mater and dura mater
   (d) dura mater and periosteum of the skull

3 Signs highly suggestive of meningitis are
   (a) headache, pyrexia, tachycardia, vomiting
   (b) pyrexia, rigors, vomiting, malaise, drowsiness, oedema
   (c) pyrexia, drowsiness, slow pulse, papilloedema, muscle spasm
   (d) headache and tachycardia plus (b)

4 The right and left cerebral hemispheres are joined by the
   (a) corpus callosum   (b) corpus luteum
   (c) pons   (d) cerebellum

5 Which one of the following consists of white matter? The
   (a) internal capsule   (b) basal ganglia
   (c) thalamus   (d) hypothalamus

6 Grey matter consists of
   (a) axons   (b) neuroglial connective tissue
   (c) peripheral nerves   (d) nerve cells

7 Intelligence, thought, reason and conscience are provided by the
   (a) hypothalamus   (b) thalamus
   (c) basal ganglia   (d) cerebral cortex

# Nervous System

8 Muscular co-ordination is controlled by the
   (a) cerebellum   (b) pyramids
   (c) thalamus     (d) parietal cortex

9 Upper motor neurons are present in the
   (a) cerebrum   (b) brain and medulla
   (c) medulla    (d) pons

10 Lower motor neurons are present in the
   (a) cerebrum   (b) cerebellum
   (c) putamen    (d) pons, medulla and spinal cord

11 A simple tendon reflex utilises only
   (a) sensory and connector neurons
   (b) sensory, connector and motor neurons
   (c) sensory, motor and cerebral neurons
   (d) cerebral neurons

12 Monoamine oxidase inhibitors are drugs which are
   (a) sedatives    (b) tranquillisers
   (c) analgesics   (d) antidepressives

13 Migraine is not treated with
   (a) aspirin    (b) ergotamine
   (c) morphine   (d) methysergide

14 A feeling of rotation is called
   (a) migraine         (b) vertigo
   (c) lightheadedness  (d) ataxia

15 Paralysis of both legs is called
   (a) hemiplegia   (b) monoplegia
   (c) paraplegia   (d) hemiparesis

16 In prolonged paralysis due to upper motor neuron damage there is not
   (a) flaccidity   (b) spasticity
   (c) clonus       (d) brisk reflexes

17 Hemiplegia cannot be due to

(a) a stroke  (b) multiple sclerosis  (c) head injury
(d) pressure on the spinal cord by a tumour of the lumbar region

18 A stroke is not due to cerebral

(a) abscess  (b) thrombosis
(c) haemorrhage  (d) embolism

19 A cerebral embolism cannot arise from clot situated in the

(a) left atrium of the heart  (b) deep veins of the leg
(c) left ventricle of the heart
(d) ascending aorta, on an ulcerated plaque of atheroma

20 The comatose patient should not lie

(a) on the left side  (b) on the right side
(c) supine  (d) prone

21 The most important of the following treatments in the unconscious patient is

(a) catheterisation  (b) enemas
(c) clear airway  (d) ripple mattress

22 The unconscious patient is not liable to

(a) photophobia  (b) dehydration
(c) pressure sores  (d) bronchopneumonia

23 A paralysed patient need not be turned if on a

(a) ripple mattress  (b) waterbed  (c) airbed
(d) the patient should be turned regularly, e.g. every two hours, irrespective of the type of mattress used

24 The partially paralysed patient should

(a) remain lying down  (b) sit up in bed
(c) stay in an armchair
(d) get up and exercise as soon as possible

# Nervous System

25 The paralysed patient who is attempting to walk should

   (a) wear well-fitting shoes   (b) wear loose slippers
   (c) use well-fitting slippers   (d) walk in bare feet

26 The patient with motor dysphasia who is trying to speak tends to get annoyed predominantly because

   (a) he is annoyed with the nurse or doctor
   (b) he does not like the hospital food
   (c) he is angry with himself for not being able to say what he wants to
   (d) he has a psychosis

27 Aneurysm refers to

   (a) subdural haematoma   (b) a swelling of an artery
   (c) a swelling of a vein   (d) any of these

28 A patient with a subarachnoid haemorrhage is nursed in

   (a) a clean and brightly lit room
   (b) a dark room and stays in bed for four to six weeks
   (c) a well-ventilated, brightly-lit room   (d) an armchair

29 Epilepsy is not due to

   (a) a genetic predisposition   (b) hyperglycaemia
   (c) head injury   (d) a brain tumour

30 Convulsions are not due to

   (a) cerebral ischaemia   (b) hypoglycaemia or uraemia
   (c) acidosis   (d) toxaemia of pregnancy

31 In a grand mal (major epilepsy) attack of average duration the patient should be

   (a) restrained and a spoon forced between the teeth
   (b) protected from injury and his collar and tie loosened
   (c) given phenobarbitone immediately
   (d) given a light anaesthetic

32 The treatment of Parkinsonism is with

   (a) levodopa or benzhexol    (b) troxidone or ethosuximide
   (c) phenobarbitone or phenytoin
   (d) chlorpromazine

33 In chorea the movements are

   (a) voluntary and regular    (b) voluntary and irregular
   (c) involuntary and regular    (d) involuntary and irregular

34 One of the following is not a cause of coma

   (a) Parkinsonism    (b) epilepsy
   (c) diabetic ketoacidosis    (d) uraemia

35 Coma is not caused by

   (a) meningitis    (b) syringomyelia
   (c) cerebral tumour    (d) hypothermia

36 Paraplegia cannot be due to

   (a) tumour pressing on the spinal cord    (b) myelitis
   (c) chorea    (d) spina bifida

37 Poliomyelitis is due to a

   (a) bacillus    (b) coccus    (c) virus    (d) fungus

38 Polyneuropathy (peripheral neuropathy) does not produce

   (a) spastic paralysis    (b) flaccid paralysis
   (c) numbness
   (d) paraesthesiae (abnormal sensations)

39 Papilloedema is

   (a) swelling around the eye    (b) swelling of the optic disc
   (c) oedema of the eyeball
   (d) oedema of the papillary muscles

40 The treatment of a subdural haematoma is

   (a) rest in bed and sedation
   (b) removal through a burr hole
   (c) intravenous mannitol    (d) hypotensive drugs

41 The psychopathic personality is

   (a) quiet and docile   (b) aggressive but responsible
   (c) quietly antisocial and responds to discipline
   (d) antisocial, irresponsible and aggressive

42 The schizophrenic is an

   (a) introvert with disturbed perception and emotion
   (b) introvert with normal perception and emotion
   (c) extrovert with normal perception and emotion
   (d) extrovert with disturbed behaviour

43 Retarded depression is least likely to be treated with

   (a) imipramine (Tofranil)
   (b) monoamine oxidase inhibitors
   (c) precautions against suicide   (d) chlorpromazine

# Answers

1 (b) The arachnoid granulations absorb cerebrospinal fluid into the venous sinuses. The brachial plexus is the nerve plexus supplying the arm.
2 (b) It lies in the subarachnoid space.
3 (c) Papilloedema and a slow pulse rate usually indicate increased intracranial pressure. Muscle spasm, e.g. neck stiffness, in the presence of papilloedema, indicates meningeal inflammation. (a), (b) or (d) may occur in many infections, although (b) is likely to be acute pyelonephritis.
4 (a) A corpus luteum is in the ovary. The pons and cerebellum lie below the cerebral hemispheres.
5 (a) The other three are areas of grey matter.
6 (d)
7 (d) The cerebral cortex contains the higher centres.

8  (a) The pyramids are tracts in the medulla which contain motor nerve fibres. The thalamus and parietal cortex are primarily concerned with sensation.
9  (a)
10 (d) The midbrain, pons and medulla contain the lower motor neurons to the cranial nerves. The spinal cord contains the lower motor neurons to the remainder of the body.
11 (b) A simple tendon reflex needs a sensory input and a motor output, joined by one or more connector neurons. It does not require the cerebrum.
12 (d)
13 (c) Migraine is a recurrent condition, morphine may, therefore, lead to addiction.
14 (b)
15 (c)
16 (a) There may be flaccidity for a few hours immediately after e.g. a stroke, but it is *not prolonged* and spasticity, clonus and brisk reflexes then appear.
17 (d) This cannot affect an arm. It may cause *para*plegia.
18 (a) A stroke is a *vascular* lesion affecting the brain.
19 (b) Emboli from deep venous thrombosis impact in the *pulmonary* arterial system.
20 (c) If the patient lies on his back, facing upwards (supine) he may inhale secretions.
21 (c) If the airway is obstructed, little else matters!
22 (a) The patient is unconscious!
23 (d)
24 (d)
25 (a) Shoes give a better balance. Slippers may be dangerous.
26 (c) He is usually annoyed with himself rather than with others. He should, therefore, be helped sympathetically, not scolded. If he has only motor dysphasia he knows what he wishes to say but is unable to say it. His intact sensory centres sense his garbled speech—to his annoyance.
27 (b) A swelling of a vein is called a varicosity.
28 (b) The patient is likely to have photophobia for the first few days.
29 (b) The other 3 choices may cause epilepsy.
30 (c)
31 (b) Restraint and force should not be used. *Immediate* sedation during a brief attack is neither practical nor necessary. Drug treatment should await investigation of the cause, and is usually not recommended for a *single* fit.

32  (a)  The other drugs are used in petit mal (b), and grand mal (c).
Chlorpromazine may produce the symptoms of Parkinsonism.
33  (d)
34  (a)  Parkinsonism is localised to the basal ganglia.
35  (b)
36  (c)  Paraplegia (paralysis of both legs) is due to damage to the spinal cord or lower motor neurons. Chorea affects the basal ganglia in the brain.
37  (c)
38  (a)  Polyneuropathy produces sensory disturbance and lower motor neuron paralysis.
Spastic paralysis is due to *upper* motor neuron damage.
39  (b)
40  (b)  It must be removed surgically.
41  (d)  He cannot be disciplined.
42  (a)
43  (d)  Chlorpromazine is more likely to be used in *agitated* depression.

# 14 Musculoskeletal System and Skin

1 How many cervical vertebrae are there?

   (a) five    (b) seven    (c) eight    (d) eleven

2 The intervertebral discs lie between adjacent vertebral

   (a) transverse processes    (b) pedicles
   (c) bodies    (d) laminae

3 How many pairs of ribs are there normally?

   (a) twelve in males and females    (b) thirteen in females
   (c) eleven in males and females    (d) eleven in males

4 The spinal cord runs

   (a) in front of the vertebral bodies    (b) behind the laminae
   (c) behind the vertebral bodies
   (d) in some other position

5 One of the following is not part of a long bone

   (a) articular cartilage    (b) shaft
   (c) head    (d) transverse process

6 The best muscles for the injection of 5 to 10 ml of irritant solution are

   (a) forearm    (b) deltoid
   (c) lower part of the glutei    (d) upper part of the glutei

7 Rheumatoid disease is a disease

   (a) which is often generalised    (b) purely of joints
   (c) of joints and skin only
   (d) of joints and bones only

# Musculoskeletal System and Skin

8 One of the following is not a treatment in rheumatoid arthritis

  (a) arthrodesis    (b) synovectomy
  (c) laminectomy    (d) tenotomy

9 One of the following is not an anti-inflammatory analgesic

  (a) prednisolone    (b) aspirin
  (c) phenylbutazone   (d) indoprofen

10 Osteoarthrosis ('osteoarthritis') is primarily

  (a) an inflammatory disorder    (b) a degenerative disorder
  (c) a disorder of uric acid metabolism
  (d) a myopathy

11 The pain caused by a prolapsed invertebral disc is usually due to

  (a) pressure on the spinal cord
  (b) pressure on vertebral bone
  (c) pressure on nerve roots or stretching of the meninges
  (d) distortion of the nucleus pulposus in the disc

12 The treatment of most patients with a prolapsed intervertebral disc is

  (a) exercises         (b) laminectomy
  (c) rest and analgesic   (d) plaster jacket

13 Pain in gout is due to

  (a) a high level of uric acid in the plasma
  (b) a low level of uric acid in the plasma
  (c) urate crystals in the bone    (d) urate crystals in the joint

14 Acute gout is treated with

  (a) phenylbutazone or colchicine
  (b) aspirin or probenecid (Benemid)
  (c) rest and sulphinpyrazone (Anturan)
  (d) neostigmine (Prostigmin)

15 One of the following is not a complication of amputation of a limb

  (a) haemorrhage    (b) polyneuritis
  (c) neuroma        (d) phantom pains

16 An autoimmune disease is a disorder in which

  (a) there is no immunity
  (b) excessive antibody production follows infection
  (c) the body produces abnormal antibodies against foreign antigen
  (d) the body produces an immune response to its own tissues

17 The outer layer of the skin consists of

  (a) dermis              (b) epidermis
  (c) subcutaneous tissue (d) fascia

18 One of the following is not a function of human skin

  (a) protection and sensation   (b) temperature regulation
  (c) production of vitamin D    (d) storage of fat

19 A small round, flat spot is called a

  (a) vesicle   (b) macule   (c) papule   (d) pustule

20 Tiny red spots of haemorrhage into the tissues are called

  (a) bruises     (b) haematomas
  (c) petechiae   (d) ecchymoses

21 Eczema is primarily

  (a) infective              (b) infective but not inflamed
  (c) infective inflammation (d) non-infective inflammation

22 Impetigo contagiosa is

  (a) a form of eczema            (b) not infective
  (c) infective but not contagious (d) contagious

23 Ringworm is infection with

  (a) worms   (b) bacteria   (c) viruses   (d) fungi

# Musculoskeletal System and Skin

24 Ringworm is spread by

   (a) direct contact and indirect contact by using combs, pillowcases or clothing used by others
   (b) direct contact only    (c) droplets    (d) infected food

25 Psoriasis is

   (a) infectious    (b) not inherited
   (c) inherited and non-infectious
   (d) infectious and inherited

26 The treatment of psoriasis is with

   (a) ultraviolet light    (b) avoidance of ultraviolet light
   (c) detergents to remove the scales
   (d) antibiotic cream

27 The treatment of epidermoid (squamous cell) carcinoma is

   (a) always excision    (b) excision or radiotherapy
   (c) medical with drugs    (d) by autosuggestion

28 Bedsores are

   (a) always due to pressure    (b) never due to pressure
   (c) gangrenous ulcers
   (d) not predisposed by sedation

# Answers

1 (b) There are seven cervical vertebrae but eight cervical nerves.
2 (c) The intervertebral discs buffer mechanical shocks transmitted through the vertebral bodies.
3 (a) Twelve pairs of ribs are present in both males and females.

4 (c)
5 (d) Transverse processes are parts of vertebrae.
6 (d) The upper and outer parts of the glutei ('buttocks'), so as to avoid the sciatic nerve.
7 (a) Rheumatoid disease affects many tissues, including joints, lungs, peripheral nerves, and blood vessels.
8 (c)
9 (a) Corticosteroids (such as prednisolone) are anti-inflammatory but are *not* analgesics.
10 (b) Osteoarthrosis is primarily a degenerative disorder, but there may be some inflammation *secondary* to joint damage.
11 (c) Pressure on the spinal cord is much less common than pressure on nerve roots and the question asks what the pain is *usually* due to.
12 (c) *Most* patients respond to rest and analgesic. A plaster jacket or laminectomy is also correct treatment—but only in a minority of patients.
13 (d)
14 (a) Probenecid and sulphinpyrazone aid the excretion of uric acid and are used between attacks, in chronic gout. They are antagonised by aspirin.
Neostigmine is used in myasthenia gravis.
15 (b)
16 (d) The body produces an immune response against its own tissues. (Auto = self).
17 (b) Epi = upon, dermis = skin.
18 (d) Storage of fat is a function of the subcutaneous tissue which is not part of the skin.
19 (b)
20 (c) Haematomas are raised, and ecchymoses are flat, bruises.
21 (d) Eczema is an inflammation but not an infection.
22 (d) It is a very contagious infection.
23 (d) Ringworm fungi (*Tinea*).
24 (a)
25 (c) The predisposition to psoriasis is inherited. It is not an infection.
26 (a) Drying substances, such as detergents, should be avoided.
27 (b) Either excision or radiotherapy gives a high cure rate.
28 (c) Sores may be due to friction, e.g. dragging a patient, who has a friable or moist skin, along the bed. They are gangrenous ulcers, i.e. ulcers due to death of skin caused by a

defective blood supply, such as prolonged pressure or a locally high pressure (creases in sheets, hard pads). Sedation makes the patient less mobile, thus predisposing to more prolonged pressure in a given position.

# 15 The Special Senses and Geriatrics

1. One of the following is not part of the wall of the eye
   (a) sclera   (b) lens   (c) choroid   (d) retina

2. Muscle fibres are present in the
   (a) choroid   (b) lens   (c) iris   (d) retina

3. The blind spot in the eye is the
   (a) optic disc   (b) macula lutea
   (c) ciliary body   (d) iris

4. The posterior chamber of the eye lies
   (a) between the cornea and iris
   (b) between the iris and lens
   (c) behind the lens   (d) in some other position

5. Mydriatic drugs
   (a) dilate the pupil   (b) constrict the pupil
   (c) are used in glaucoma   (d) both (b) and (c)

6. A drug used to treat glaucoma is
   (a) atropine   (b) homatropine
   (c) pilocarpine   (d) cyclopentolate

7. Blindness is rarely caused by
   (a) trachoma   (b) glaucoma
   (c) cataract   (d) allergic conjunctivitis

8. One of the following is not a primary sensation of taste
   (a) sweet   (b) salt   (c) musty   (d) bitter

# The Special Senses and Geriatrics

9  The external auditory canal contains ceruminous glands which secrete

   (a) mucus   (b) wax   (c) sweat   (d) serum

10 The ear transmits postural impulses from the semicircular canals to the

   (a) cerebrum      (b) temporal lobe
   (c) cerebellum    (d) auditory ossicles

11 Nerve deafness is not due to

   (a) otitis media            (b) congenital rubella
   (c) persistent loud sound   (d) streptomycin

12 Otitis media is usually due to spread of infection from the

   (a) external auditory meatus   (b) pharynx
   (c) blood                      (d) mastoid

13 If pus is present in the middle ear in otitis media the treatment is

   (a) myringotomy and antibiotic   (b) antibiotic alone
   (c) myringotomy alone            (d) mastoidectomy

14 The elderly are more liable than young people to suffer from

   (a) rheumatic fever    (b) malnutrition
   (c) acute leukaemia    (d) glandular fever

15 The elderly do not commonly suffer from

   (a) osteoarthrosis   (b) constipation
   (c) osteoporosis     (d) haemophilia

16 The incidence of deficiency disorders in the elderly is

   (a) low   (b) high
   (c) the same as in young adults
   (d) the same as in middle age

17 The assessment of an elderly person should include

   (a) physical abilities   (b) faculties
   (c) continence           (d) all of these

18 If an elderly person falls easily in the dark or tends to slip on polished floors and to be accident prone, he should be
   (a) confined to bed for his own safety
   (b) confined to a chair
   (c) allowed to continue as usual
   (d) treated in some other way

# Answers

1 (b)
2 (c) The iris contains circular and radiating muscle fibres which control the size of the pupil.
3 (a)
4 (b) The posterior chamber of the eye does *not* refer to that part containing vitreous humour.
5 (a) Mydriatics dilate the pupil (but may precipitate glaucoma).
6 (c) Pilocarpine (a miotic drug) constricts the pupil thus improving drainage of aqueous humour into the canal of Schlemm.
7 (d) Allergic conjunctivitis does not cause blindness so long as complications do not arise.
8 (c) 'Musty' is a sensation of smell.
9 (b) Ceruminous glands secrete wax.
10 (c) The cerebellum receives information concerning the position of the head, muscles and joints so as to co-ordinate body balance.
11 (a) Otitis media may lead to *conduction* deafness, not nerve deafness.
12 (b) Infection usually spreads along the Eustachian tube from the pharynx.
13 (a) Myringotomy (making an opening in the eardrum) will drain pus from the middle ear. Mastoidectomy is only neces-

# The Special Senses and Geriatrics

sary if mastoiditis complicates otitis media, but the question did not ask about this.
14 (b) Rheumatic fever, acute leukaemia and glandular fever predominantly affect children and young adults.
15 (d) Haemophilia is an uncommon condition, and many haemophiliacs die before reaching old age.
16 (b)
17 (d)
18 (d) He should *not* be confined to bed or to a chair since this leads to a permanently incapacitated state, contractures and apathy. He should be provided with aids such as non-slip mats instead of polished floors, fireguards, etc., and receive help from the social services.

# Matching Block Questions

An example of this style of question is:

Match each sign with its meaning

1 Aphasia    2 Dyslexia    3 Ataxia    4 Vertigo
A A feeling of rotation
B Inability to speak
C Difficulty in reading
D Inco-ordination

| 1 | 2 | 3 | 4 |
|---|---|---|---|
| B | C | D | A |

4 marks

1  Match each drug with its action

    1 Aminophylline    2 Tolbutamide    3 Codeine    4 Nitrazepam
    A Analgesic
    B Sedation
    C Dilatation of veins
    D Lowered blood glucose level

| 1 | 2 | 3 | 4 |
|---|---|---|---|
|   |   |   |   |

2  Match each drug with its dose

    1 Digoxin    2 Morphine    3 Heparin    4 Tetracycline
    A 15 mg
    B 250
    C 0.25 mg
    D 100 mg

| 1 | 2 | 3 | 4 |
|---|---|---|---|
|   |   |   |   |

3  Match each symptom with its cause

    1 Colic    2 Haemoptysis    3 Goitre    4 Gangrene
    A Arterial embolism
    B Mitral stenosis
    C Stone
    D Iodine deficiency

| 1 | 2 | 3 | 4 |
|---|---|---|---|
|   |   |   |   |

# Matching Block Questions

4 Match each disorder with its treatment

   1. Chronic bronchitis    2 Pleural effusion
   3 Pulmonary oedema    4 Pleurisy
   A Paracentesis
   B Analgesic
   C 60% oxygen
   D 30% oxygen

| 1 | 2 | 3 | 4 |
|---|---|---|---|
|   |   |   |   |

5 Match each disorder with its cause

   1 'Hay fever'    2 Cystic fibrosis
   3 Carcinoma of the bronchus    4 Pneumoconiosis
   A Cigarette smoking
   B Allergy to pollen and other particles
   C Mineral dusts
   D Viscid glandular secretions

| 1 | 2 | 3 | 4 |
|---|---|---|---|
|   |   |   |   |

6 Match each disorder with the symptom

   1 Myocardial infarction    2 Peptic ulcer    3 Pneumonia
   4 Pleurisy
   A Epigastric pain, relieved by milk
   B Stabbing pain on breathing
   C Dyspnoea and cyanosis
   D Retrosternal pain and shock

| 1 | 2 | 3 | 4 |
|---|---|---|---|
|   |   |   |   |

7 Match the disorder with the investigation

   1 Jaundice    2 Myocardial infarction
   3 Carcinoma of the colon    4 Pneumonia
   A Faeces for occult blood
   B Serum alkaline phosphatase and transaminase
   C White blood cell count
   D Serum transaminase and electrocardiography

| 1 | 2 | 3 | 4 |
|---|---|---|---|
|   |   |   |   |

8 Match the organ with its function

   1 Liver   2 Pancreas   3 Gall bladder   4 Stomach
   A Secretion of trypsinogen
   B Secretion of pepsinogen
   C Storage of bile
   D Formation of bile

   | 1 | 2 | 3 | 4 |
   |---|---|---|---|
   |   |   |   |   |

9 Match the observation with its cause

   1 Retention of urine   2 Anuria   3 Polyuria
   4 Glycosuria
   A Acute renal failure
   B Low renal threshold for glucose
   C Prostatic enlargement*
   D Chronic renal failure

   | 1 | 2 | 3 | 4 |
   |---|---|---|---|
   |   |   |   |   |

10 Match the disease with its treatment

   1 Hypertension   2 Asthma   3 Diverticulitis
   4 Venous thrombosis
   A Diuretic and propranolol
   B Sympathomimetic e.g. orciprenaline
   C Antibiotic
   D Anticoagulant

   | 1 | 2 | 3 | 4 |
   |---|---|---|---|
   |   |   |   |   |

# Answers

| 1 | 1C | 2D | 3A | 4B |
| 2 | 1C | 2A | 3D | 4B |
| 3 | 1C | 2B | 3D | 4A |
| 4 | 1D | 2A | 3C | 4B |
| 5 | 1B | 2D | 3A | 4C |
| 6 | 1D | 2A | 3C | 4B |

# Matching Block Questions

| | | | | |
|---|---|---|---|---|
| 7 | 1B | 2D | 3A | 4C |
| 8 | 1D | 2A | 3C | 4B |
| 9 | 1C | 2A | 3D | 4B |
| 10 | 1A | 2B | 3C | 4D |